# Virginia Campground Locator Map

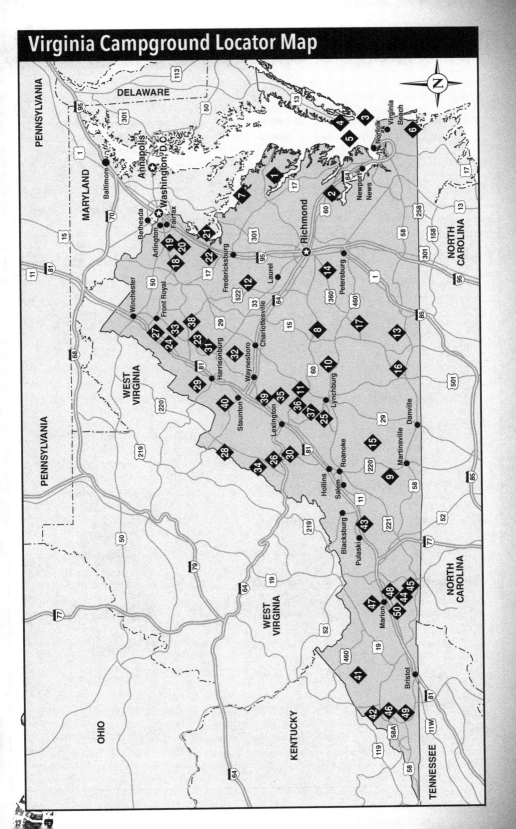

# Virginia Campground Map Legend

 **North indicator**

**➡** **Off-map or pinpoint-indication arrow**

**△** **Campground name and location**

**▲¹ ⌂ ⌂ ⌐** **Individual tents, cottages, cabins, and lean-tos within campground area**

---

**△** **Group site**

**Richmond ✪ Capital**

**Lynchburg ○ City or town**

**NATIONAL FOREST STATE PARK** **Public lands**

**Main Trail - - - - - Hiking trails**

**▥ Steps**

---

**━━64━━** **Interstate highways**

**━58━** **US highways**

**━(347)━** **State roads**

**Quail Rd. FT 352 FR 603** **Other roads**

---

**- - - - - - - Dirt/gravel roads**

**- ·· - ·· - ·· - Area boundary**

**Potomac River River or stream**

**Lake Lake or pond**

---

| | | | | | |
|---|---|---|---|---|---|
| ⌶ | Bridge or tunnel | ⚲ | Playground | ⅋ | Picnic area |
| ♨ | Amphitheater | P | Parking | 🏕 | Sheltered picnic area |
| ⛲ | Water access | 🚤 | Marina or boat ramp | ⛏ | Lodge |
| ♿ | Wheelchair accessible | ⬛ | Laundry | 🎣 | Fishing area |
| 🚻 | Restroom | ℭ | Telephone | 🚿 | Showers |
| ⚇ | Pit toilet | 🏇 | Equestrian site | 🚏 | Dump station |
| 🛒 | Store | $ | Pay station | 🏃 | Baseball field |
| 🚮 | Trash disposal | 🏊 | Swimming | 🏹 | Shooting range |
| ▲ | Overlook | ⌂ | Ranger station | 🏌 | Frisbee golf |
| ☂ | Beach | 🔥 | Firewood | ♻ | Recycling bin |
| 🍴 | Dining | 🚫 | No swimming | ⊞ | First aid |
| ⊘ | Information | ⚱ | Fire pit | ◈ | Appalachian Trail |
| ⒸVending | | | | | |

# OVERVIEW MAP KEY

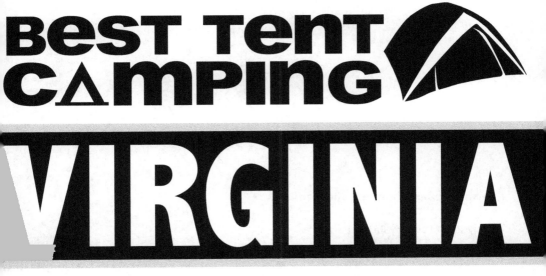

# BEST TENT CAMPING

# VIRGINIA

## YOUR CAR-CAMPING GUIDE TO SCENIC BEAUTY, THE SOUNDS OF NATURE, AND AN ESCAPE FROM CIVILIZATION

3rd Edition

# RANDY PORTER

MENASHA RIDGE PRESS
*Your Guide to the Outdoors Since 1982*

**⁝⁝** *I'd like to dedicate this revised edition to my Sweet Melissa, who shared her time, her energy, and her love to help me complete this guide and enjoy every moment together doing so.*

**Best Tent Camping: Virginia, 3rd Edition**

Copyright © 2014 by Randy Porter
All rights reserved
Published by Menasha Ridge Press
Distributed by Publishers Group West
Third edition, first printing

CATALOGING-IN-PUBLICATION DATA IS AVAILABLE FROM THE LIBRARY OF CONGRESS

ISBN 9780897325066 (pbk.) — ISBN 9780897325073 (ebook)
ISBN 9781634042048 (hardcover)

Cover design by Scott McGrew
Cover photo by Pat & Chuck Blackley / Alamy
Text design by Annie Long
Cartography by Steve Jones and Scott McGrew
Indexing by Ann Cassar

**MENASHA RIDGE PRESS**
An imprint of AdventureKEEN
2204 First Avenue South, Suite 102
Birmingham, Alabama 35233
**menasharidge.com**

# CONTENTS

• • • • • • • • • • • • • • • • • • • • •

## :: WESTERN VIRGINIA   79

## :: SOUTHWEST VIRGINIA   135

## :: APPENDIXES   167

# BEST CAMPGROUNDS

## :: BEST FOR SPACIOUS CAMPSITES

## :: BEST FOR SWIMMING

## :: BEST FOR WATERFALLS

# ACKNOWLEDGMENTS

● ● ● ● ● ● ● ● ● ● ● ● ● ● ● ● ● ● ● ● ● ● ● ●

**T**hanks to all those who work to keep Virginia's parks and wild areas crown jewels of the commonwealth. In particular, I'd like to thank the following, who responded to my request for updated information: Shawn Callahan, City of Chesapeake Parks and Recreation; Daniel Jordan, Kiptopeke State Park; Zoe Rogers, Virginia Department of Recreation and Conservation; Laura Moss, Bear Creek Lake State Park; Barbara Miller, James River State Park; Bill Crawford, James River State Park; Stephanie Allen, Staunton River State Park; Fairy Stone State Park; Tracy Ballesteros, Prince William Forest Park; Ann Cole, Bull Run Regional Park; Todd Benson, Pohick Bay Regional Park; Hazel Mehne, Shenandoah National Park; Wayne Nicely, Lake Robertson Recreation Area; Stephanie Chapman, Lee Ranger District of the George Washington and Jefferson National Forests; Kathryn Hall, Glenwood-Pedlar Ranger District of the George Washington and Jefferson National Forests; Dawn Coulson, Warm Springs Ranger District of the George Washington and Jefferson National Forests; Mike Bodkin, Warm Springs Ranger District of the George Washington and Jefferson National Forests; Claytor Lake State Park; Mount Rogers Recreation Area of the George Washington and Jefferson National Forests; Theresa Tibbs, Grayson Highlands State Park; Camp Hosts Bob and Peg Penater.

# PREFACE

● ● ● ● ● ● ● ● ● ● ● ● ● ● ● ● ● ● ● ● ● ● ●

**V**irginia is a state, actually a commonwealth, whose history and natural beauty are best described in superlatives. Her scenery varies from the coastal plain along the Atlantic Ocean and Chesapeake Bay to mountain ranges in the west and southwest. Her history parallels that of the New World, with the first settlers arriving in 1607, more U.S. presidents coming from Virginia than any other state, and the majority of Civil War battles being fought here. While the country was mired in the Great Depression in the 1930s, Virginia's public lands were the fortunate recipients of much of the labor of the Civilian Conservation Corps. As you travel about through the Old Dominion's federal- and state-managed public lands, you'll swim in lakes, hike on trails, and pitch your tent in areas that were born of one of the country's darkest periods.

I've lived in Virginia and explored its wooded countryside for more than four decades, and I still find myself overwhelmed by her glorious landscape and central role in the birth and growth of the United States. There's no better way to get to know the Old Dominion than by pitching a tent and camping out up close and personal. Walk her trails, fish in her streams, and sleep under her stars, and I'm convinced that you, too, will be taken by her charms.

# INTRODUCTION

## How to Use This Guidebook

**The publishers of Menasha Ridge Press** welcome you to *Best Tent Camping: Virginia*. Whether you're new to this activity or you've been sleeping in your portable outdoor shelter over decades of outdoor adventures, please review the following information. It explains how we have worked with the author to organize this book and how you can make the best use of it.

Some passages in this introduction are applicable to all of the books in the Best Tent Camping guidebook series. Where this isn't the case, such as in the descriptions of weather, wildlife, and plants, the author has provided information specific to your area.

### :: THE RATINGS & RATING CATEGORIES

As with all of the books in the publisher's Best Tent Camping series, this guidebook's author personally experienced dozens of campgrounds and campsites to select the top 50 locations in this region. Within that universe of 50 sites, the author then ranked each one in the six categories described below. Each campground in this guidebook is superlative in its own way. For example, a site may be rated only one star in one category but perhaps five stars in another category. This rating system allows you to choose your destination based on the attributes that are most important to you. Though these ratings are subjective, they're still excellent guidelines for finding the perfect camping experience for you and your companions. Below and following we describe the criteria for each of the attributes in our five-star rating system:

★ ★ ★ ★ ★    The site is **ideal** in that category.

★ ★ ★ ★    The site is **exemplary** in that category.

★ ★ ★    The site is **very good** in that category.

★ ★    The site is **above average** in that category.

★    The site is **acceptable** in that category.

### *Beauty*

If this category needs explanation at all, it is simply to say that the true beauty of a campground lies not just in what you can see but also in what you can't see. Or hear. Like a freeway. Or roaring motorboats. Or the crack, pop, pop, boom of a rifle range. An equally important factor for me on the beauty scale is the condition of the campground itself and to what extent it has been left in its natural state. Beauty also, of course, takes into consideration any fabulous views of mountains, water, or other natural phenomena.

### *Privacy*

No one who enjoys the simplicity of tent camping wants to be walled in on all sides by RVs the size of tractor-trailers. This category goes hand in hand with the previous one because part of the beauty of a campsite has to do with the privacy of its surroundings. If you've ever crawled out of your tent to embrace a stunning summer morning in your skivvies and found several pairs of very curious eyes staring at you from the neighbor's picture window, you'll know what I mean. I look for campsites that are graciously spaced with lots of heavy foliage in between. You usually have to drive or even hike a little deeper into the campground complex for these.

## Spaciousness

This is the category you toss the coin on—and keep your fingers crossed. I'm not as much of a stickler for this category because I'm happy if there's room to park the car off the main campground road, enough space to pitch a two- or four-man tent in a reasonably flat and dry spot, a picnic table for meal preparation, and a fire pit safely away from the tenting area. At most campgrounds, site spaciousness is sacrificed for site privacy and vice versa. Sometimes you get extremely lucky and have both. Don't be greedy.

## Quiet

Again, this category goes along with the beauty of a place. When I go camping, I want to hear the sounds of nature. You know: birds chirping, the wind sighing, a surf crashing, a brook babbling. It's not always possible to control the volume of your fellow campers, so the closer you can get to natural sounds that can drown them out, the better. Actually, when you have a chance to listen to the quiet of nature, you'll find that it is really rather noisy. But what a lovely cacophony!

## Security

Quite a few of the campgrounds in this book are in remote and primitive places without on-site security patrol. In essence, you're on your own. Common sense is a great asset in these cases. Don't leave expensive outdoor gear or valuable camera equipment lying around your campsite or even within view inside your car. If you are at a hosted site, you may feel more comfortable leaving valuables with them. Or let them know you'll be gone for an extended period so they can keep an eye on your things.

Unfortunately, even in lightly camped areas, vandalism is a common problem. In many places, the wild animals can do as much damage as humans. If you leave food inside your tent or around the campsite, don't be surprised if things look slightly ransacked when you return. The most frequent visitors to food-strewn campsites are birds, squirrels, chipmunks, deer, and bears.

## Cleanliness

By and large, the campgrounds in this book rank well in this category. I think Virginia campgrounds are some of the cleanest and tidiest spots I've been in, due to the fine management of park and Forest Service attendants. The only time they tend to fall a bit short of expectations is on busy summer weekends. This is usually only in the larger, more developed compounds. In more remote areas, the level of cleanliness is most often dependent on the good habits of the campers themselves. Keep that in mind wherever you camp.

## :: THE CAMPGROUND PROFILE

Each profile contains a concise but informative narrative of the campground and individual sites. Not only is the property described, but also readers can get a general idea of the recreational opportunities available—what's in the area and perhaps suggestions for touristy activities. This descriptive text is enhanced with three helpful sidebars: Ratings, Key Information, and Getting There (accurate driving directions that lead you to the campground from the nearest major roadway, along with GPS coordinates).

## :: THE OVERVIEW MAP, MAP KEY, AND LEGEND

Use the overview map on the inside front cover to assess the exact location of each campground. The campground's number appears not only on the overview map but also on the map key facing the overview map, in the table of contents, and on the profile's first page. This book is organized by region, as indicated in the table of contents.

A map legend that details the symbols found on the campground-layout maps appears on the inside back cover.

## :: CAMPGROUND-LAYOUT MAPS

Each profile includes a detailed map of campground sites, internal roads, facilities, and other key items.

## :: GPS CAMPGROUND-ENTRANCE COORDINATES

Readers can easily access all campgrounds in this book by using the directions given and the overview map, which shows at least one major road leading into the area. But for those who enjoy using GPS technology to navigate, the book includes coordinates for each campground's entrance in latitude and longitude, expressed in degrees and decimal minutes.

**GPS COORDINATES:**   N37° 46.973′   W76° 34.780′

To convert GPS coordinates from degrees, minutes, and seconds to the above degrees–decimal minutes format, the seconds are divided by 60. For more on GPS technology, visit **usgs.gov.**

*A note of caution:* Actual GPS devices will easily guide you to any of these campgrounds, but users of smartphone mapping apps will find that cell phone service is often unavailable in the hills and hollows where many of these hideaways are located.

# About This Book

**Virginia's history, varied topography,** and natural features are rivaled by few other states. As I crisscrossed its length and breadth, I never ceased to be fascinated by those attributes. Just as varied are the places to camp. Some parts of the state have changed little since the country's first settlers stepped ashore in 1607, and others would be unrecognizable by John Smith and his fellows. For that matter, some areas appeared foreign to me when I revisited several years later.

As you travel with *Best Tent Camping: Virginia* in hand, I know that you, too, will be mesmerized by a state whose camping areas vary so markedly from one another. From the coast to the tops of mountains, and from large urban areas to the great beyond, I found a lot of great places to pitch a tent for a night or longer. If there were but 50 campgrounds in the entire Old Dominion, as the Commonwealth of Virginia is often called, my task would have been much simpler. I found vast differences, from municipal campgrounds in northern Virginia to primitive ones in the national forests. Depending on where you choose to sleep, you may find yourself next to a golf course or you may find nary a pit toilet.

The question then arises: "What's camping all about if so many different sites can fall under one title?" Is it finding wilderness among a population center of 3 million people, or is it looking into the flames of a fire that's miles from the nearest person? I'm not sure that one definition fits all, nor would I be comfortable with a policy that would arbitrarily rule out some and include others.

Ultimately, camping is not about the size of your tent, the distance from the next site, or even what sanitary facilities are there, although those things are definitely good to know. It's about the mindset that you bring to the outdoors and the one you leave at home. But this I guarantee—if you embark into the outdoors with an open mind and a spirit of adventure, wherever you go in the woods, you'll find yourself at home. You'll learn a little about your surroundings and a lot about yourself.

## :: WEATHER

Virginia offers four distinct seasons, although Mother Nature sometimes gets them confused. In short, year-round camping is a real possibility, but extreme winter weather will be more likely and severe as one travels west. Winter camping in far Southwest Virginia, in particular, can be very cold, but it's also the coolest region in other seasons. Summer is often hot and humid along Virginia's coastal region, but the rivers, swimming holes, and lakes at most campgrounds keep campers comfortable in even the worst heat wave. Spring and fall are beautiful times to be outdoors in Virginia. In the spring, wildflowers are abundant, dogwood and redwood blooms brighten the gray forest, turkeys gobble in the early morning, and spring peepers serenade you from the lakes and streams near camp. Fall in the mountains is nearly everyone's favorite camping season. Cold frosty mornings chip away at the lassitude left from summer's heat. In fall's crisp air you begin breathing easily and deeply for the first time in months, and your body wakes up ready to hit the trails. Pleasing hues of orange, red, yellow, and caramel decorate the forest as the trees prepare to shed their summer foliage. Additional benefits of autumn camping are the absence of humidity, heat, bugs, and crowds; the streams are shallow and easier to cross; and the bare trees open up scenic views obscured by lush foliage during the warmer months.

## :: FIRST-AID KIT

A useful first-aid kit may contain more items than you might think necessary. These are just the basics. Prepackaged kits in waterproof bags (Atwater Carey and Adventure Medical make them) are available. As a preventive measure, take along sunscreen and insect repellent. Even though quite a few items are listed here, they pack down into a small space:

- Ace bandages or Spenco joint wraps
- Adhesive bandages, such as Band-Aids
- Antibiotic ointment (Neosporin or the generic equivalent)
- Antiseptic or disinfectant, such as Betadine or hydrogen peroxide
- Aspirin, acetaminophen, or ibuprofen
- Benadryl or the generic equivalent, diphenhydramine (in case of allergic reactions)
- Butterfly-closure bandages
- Comb and tweezers (for removing ticks from your skin)
- Epinephrine in a prefilled syringe (for severe allergic reactions to such things as beestings)
- Gauze (one roll and six 4-by-4-inch compress pads
- LED flashlight or headlamp
- Matches or lighter
- Moist towelettes
- Moleskin/Spenco 2nd Skin
- Pocketknife or multipurpose tool
- Waterproof first-aid tape
- Whistle (it's more effective in signaling rescuers than your voice)

## :: ANIMAL AND PLANT HAZARDS

### Bears

*Ursus Americanus*, the American Black Bear, was reintroduced into Arkansas around 1960. They are not uncommon in Virginia's western mountains, especially in Shenandoah National Park and the George Washington and Jefferson National Forests. Normal precautions for keeping nuisance animals, such as raccoons and opossums, out of your food supply are usually all that's necessary when camping. Check campground bulletin boards when you pull into camp—there will be a notice posted if recent bear activity has occurred in the camp or its surrounding area, along with additional precautions you should take. In areas with high bear activity, be sure to use specially designed food containers. Never keep food in your tent.

### Emerald Ash Borer

Virginia's forests are under attack from the Emerald Ash Borer (EAB) and several other boring insects, so the following notice from the Virginia Department of Conservation and Recreation should be heeded at all campgrounds throughout the commonwealth.

"One of the most important things we can do to protect Virginia's trees and forest diversity is stop moving firewood. New infestations of tree-killing insects and diseases are often first found in campgrounds and parks. Why? Because people have accidentally spread invasive species when they brought firewood along with them. There are numerous Virginia counties under quarantines, issued by the Virginia Department of Agriculture and Consumer Services, due to an invasive insect pest or disease. These quarantines restrict the movement of firewood or wood by products from certain tree species. Moving firewood in violation of a quarantine is a class 1 misdemeanor and upon conviction, you could be subject to confinement in jail for up to twelve months and a fine of $2,500.00 or both."

### Poison Ivy

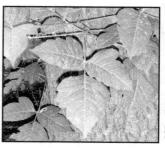

This little villain is common throughout Virginia. Watch for its three-leaf configuration, both in ground cover and vines on trees near your campsite. Within 14 hours of exposure, you'll have blisters and a terrible itch in the affected area. Wash and dry the area thoroughly with alcohol, soap, and cold water as soon as possible after exposure. Wearing long pants and sleeves will help protect you, but be careful—touching your clothing or even pets or camping gear that have contacted poison ivy may spread the plant's rash-producing oil onto your skin. If you're sensitive to the ivy's effects, bring along one of the various over-the-counter products that alleviate poison ivy's irritating symptoms.

### Snakes

Venomous snakes aren't a huge problem in Virginia, but they're out there. Copperheads are the most common. Timber rattlesnakes are occasionally sighted in the western mountains. Once while mountain biking I found myself sharing a resting spot for 15 minutes about three feet from a timber rattler. You may spot cottonmouth water moccasins in streams, lakes, and even in pools along trails in the campgrounds that are east of the I-95 corridor. Unless

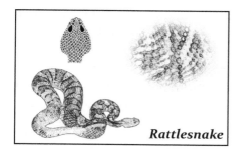

*Rattlesnake*

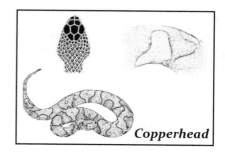

*Copperhead*

they're torpid from cold weather, snakes will see you or sense your footfalls before you reach them and move away.

## *Ticks*

Ticks are ubiquitous throughout Virginia, especially in warmer months. You can contract Lyme disease and Rocky Mountain spotted fever from these annoying little critters, but it rarely happens, especially if you're vigilant and remove them soon after they find you. Wearing light-colored clothing makes them easier to spot, and an insect repellent with DEET helps keep them away. Ticks prefer places where they're held tightly against your skin, such as elastic on socks and underwear, your underarms, waistband, and back of the knee. Tweezers are ideal for removing a tick that has already attached—just grab it as close to the skin surface as possible and firmly pull it loose without crushing it. Expect a bit of redness and itching for a few days around the bite site.

### :: CAMPING ETIQUETTE

Here are a few tips on how to create good vibes with fellow campers and wildlife you encounter.

- Make sure that you check in, pay your fee, and mark your site as directed. Don't make the mistake of grabbing a seemingly empty site that looks more appealing than your site. It could be reserved. If you're unhappy with the site you've selected, check with the campground host for other options.

- Be sensitive to the ground beneath you. Place all garbage in designated receptacles or pack it out if none is available. No one likes to see the trash that someone else has left behind.

- It's common for animals to wander through campsites, where they may be accustomed to the presence of humans (and our food). An unannounced approach, a sudden movement, or a loud noise startles most animals. A surprised animal can be dangerous to you, to others, and to themselves. Give them plenty of space.

- Plan ahead. Know your equipment, your ability, and the area where you are camping—and prepare accordingly. Be self-sufficient at all times; carry necessary supplies for changes in weather or other conditions. A well-executed trip is a satisfaction to you and to others.

- Be courteous to other campers, hikers, bikers, and anyone else you encounter.

- Strictly follow the campground's rules regarding the building of fires. Never burn trash. Trash smoke smells horrible, and trash debris in a fire pit or grill is unsightly.

- Everyone likes a fire, but bringing your own firewood from home is now forbidden by most campground operators. Bringing in wood from out of the area could introduce pests that are harmful to the forest. Use deadfall found near your campsite or purchase wood at the camp store.

## :: HAPPY CAMPING

There is nothing worse than a bad camping trip, especially because it is so easy to have a great time. To assist with making your outing a happy one, here are some pointers.

Reserve your site in advance, especially if it's a weekend or a holiday, or if the campground is wildly popular. Many prime campgrounds require at least a six-month lead time on reservations. Check before you go.

- Pick your camping buddies wisely. A family trip is pretty straightforward, but you may want to reconsider including grumpy Uncle Fred, who doesn't like bugs, sunshine, or marshmallows. After you know who's going, make sure that everyone is on the same page regarding expectations of difficulty (amenities or the lack thereof, physical exertion, and so on), sleeping arrangements, and food requirements.

- Don't duplicate equipment, such as cooking pots and lanterns, among campers in your party. Carry what you need to have a good time, but don't turn the trip into a cross-country moving experience.

- Dress for the season. Educate yourself on the temperature highs and lows of the specific part of the state you plan to visit. It may be warm at night in the summer in your backyard, but up in the mountains it will be quite chilly.

- Pitch your tent on a level surface, preferably one covered with leaves, pine straw, or grass. Use a tarp or specially designed footprint to thwart ground moisture and to protect the tent floor. Do a little site maintenance, such as picking up the small rocks and sticks that can damage your tent floor and make sleep uncomfortable. If you have a separate tent rain fly but don't think you'll need it, keep it rolled up at the base of the tent in case it starts raining at midnight.

- Consider taking a sleeping pad if the ground makes you uncomfortable. Choose a pad that is full-length and thicker than you think you might need. This will not only keep your hips from aching on hard ground, but it will also help keep you warm. A wide range of thin, light, or inflatable pads is available at camping stores today, and these are a much better choice than home air mattresses, which conduct heat away from the body and tend to deflate during the night.

- If you are not hiking in to a primitive campsite, there is no real need to skimp on food due to weight. Plan tasty meals and bring everything you will need to prepare, cook, eat, and clean up.

- If you tend to use the bathroom multiple times at night, you should plan ahead. Leaving a warm sleeping bag and stumbling around in the dark to find the restroom—whether it be a pit toilet, a fully plumbed comfort station, or just the woods—is not fun. Keep a flashlight and any other accoutrements you may need by the tent door and know exactly where to head in the dark.

- Standing dead trees and storm-damaged living trees can pose a real hazard to tent campers (foresters call these widow-makers for obvious reasons.) These trees may have loose or broken limbs that could fall at any time. When choosing a campsite or even just a spot to rest during a hike, look up.

# Coastal Virginia

# 1

# Belle Isle State Park

*The diverse ecology at Belle Isle provides a fertile environment for various birds of prey, such as bald eagles, osprey, and hawks, as well as deer, wild turkeys, and reptiles and amphibians.*

**B**elle Isle State Park lies in Virginia's Northern Neck, and its 733 acres represent a rare piece of public land on the lower Rappahannock River. (It should not be confused with the island that lies in the James River in Richmond.) The "beautiful island" itself is very spread out with large cultivated fields and coastal woodlands/swamp/wetlands separating it from developed sections. This diverse ecology provides a fertile environment for various birds of prey, such as bald eagles, osprey, and hawks, as well as deer, wild turkeys, and reptiles and amphibians. The Bay Seafood Festival in early September is one of the park's popular draws, but other programs capitalize on the natural and historical aspects. In addition to free monthly music concerts in summer, you'll also be able to participate in Native Knowledge Canoe Trip, If You Lived During the Civil War, and the Full Moon Kayak Trip. The several miles of trails that crisscross Belle Isle State Park are best enjoyed on foot. Being so close to sea level, it requires a pretty healthy dry spell for

these fields and trails to make cycling doable. However, I would recommend bringing bikes to ride on the park roads, which are wide, flat, and very lightly traveled.

The Bel Air mansion and guesthouse are the centerpiece of this park. Built in 1942 and designed by John Waterman, a former architectural historian with Colonial Williamsburg, these buildings were the home of Mr. and Mrs. John Garland Pollard Jr. They were built and decorated with the special attention characteristic of Colonial Williamsburg and were placed on the National Register of Historic Places in 1971. Pollard's father was a former governor of Virginia, was a professor at the College of William and Mary, and worked with the original restoration of Williamsburg. Both buildings are available to rent for special events like weddings, reunions, and picnics.

Kayakers and canoeists will find a quiet spot to launch their boats onto Mulberry Creek at the end of Creek Landing Road next to the 0.1-mile Fishing Creek Access boardwalk trail. Those with motorboats can launch onto Deep Creek from the southeast end of Creek Landing Road.

All 28 campsites have both water and electric hookups and are laid out along both sides of the campground loop road. They share a fairly new bathhouse, which includes laundry facilities. Sites are level with a pea gravel surface, so tent campers will find

## :: Ratings

BEAUTY: ★ ★ ★
SITE PRIVACY: ★ ★
SPACIOUSNESS: ★ ★ ★
QUIET: ★ ★ ★
SECURITY: ★ ★ ★
CLEANLINESS: ★ ★ ★

# :: Key Information

**ADDRESS:** 1632 Belle Isle Road, Lancaster, VA 22503

**OPERATED BY:** Virginia Department of Conservation and Recreation

**CONTACT:** 804-462-5030; dcr.virginia.gov

**OPEN:** March 1–early December

**SITES:** 28

**SITE AMENITIES:** Picnic table, fire ring, lantern pole, electric/water hookups

**ASSIGNMENT:** First come, first served

**REGISTRATION:** Call 800-933-PARK, visit reserveamerica.com, or on arrival; reservations highly recommended

**FACILITIES:** Water, hot showers, laundry, camp store, pay phone

**PARKING:** 2 vehicles per site in addition to camping unit

**FEE:** $27 per night

**ELEVATION:** Sea level

**RESTRICTIONS:**
- **Pets:** On leash or in enclosed area; in swimming areas on leash with overnight guests only
- **Fires:** In fire rings, stoves, or grills only
- **Alcohol:** Prohibited except inside camping units
- **Vehicles:** Up to 45 feet
- **Other:** Do not damage any trees; no motorized vehicles on trails; maximum stay is 14 days in a 30-day period; quiet hours 10 p.m.–6 a.m.

sleeping pads and under-tent ground covers to be the order of the day. Most campsites are fairly open, which is a good thing when you're this close to sea level, and mosquitoes can be an issue. Another camping option for canoeists and kayakers who don't mind roughing it is the canoe camping facility on the shoreline near the mouth of Mulberry Creek. It offers four canoe-accessible campsites and a pit privy.

The closest grocery store is a bit of a drive, so campers should plan to bring adequate provisions to cover their stay. However, Lancaster County has a lot to offer canoeists and kayakers who would like to explore other nearby waterways. Likewise, road cyclists who want to up their

mileage outside the park roads and trails may want to check out the county's flat back roads. Those who want to learn more about local goings-on should check out the county website and may want to plan their trip accordingly: **tlcva.com/things-to-do /events.** Nature lovers will want to explore nearby destinations, such as the Rappahannock River Valley National Wildlife Refuge (**fws.gov/refuge/rappahannock_river_ valley**), Chilton Woods State Forest, Hickory Hollow Natural Area Preserve, Bush Mill Stream Natural Area Preserve, Hughlett Point Natural Area Preserve, and Dameron Marsh Natural Area Preserve, as well. On the other hand, most will find Belle Isle State Park to be a great getaway.

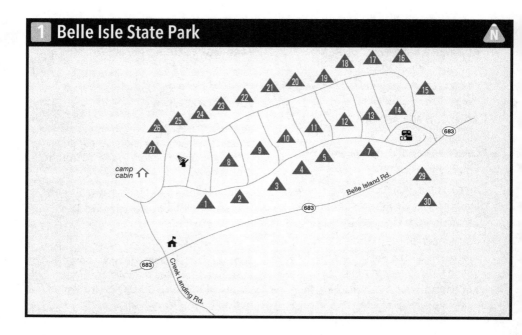

## :: Getting There

From Warsaw, take VA 3 east to VA 354. Turn right and follow it for 3 miles. Turn right onto VA 683 at Somers to the park entrance. From Kilmarnock, take VA 3 west to Lively, then turn left on VA 201 and follow it 3 miles. Turn right on VA 354, travel 3 miles, then turn left onto 683 to the park entrance.

**GPS COORDINATES** N37° 46.973 W76° 34.780

# 2

# Chippokes Plantation State Park

*Bird-watchers, history buffs, and those who enjoy outdoor recreation will find a haven on the quiet side of the James River.*

**C**hippokes Plantation State Park is located just across the James River from Jamestown, site of the first European permanent settlement in the New World. The land dates from 1619 and is one of the oldest continuously farmed properties in the United States, but the campground has only been open since 1998. The park's Farm and Forestry Museum displays thousands of artifacts, including a bull-tongue plow from the early 1600s. Exhibits show the various stages of farming, such as preparing the soil, planting, cultivating, and harvesting, as well as the related tasks of the blacksmith, wheelwright, cooper, and cobbler. The theme is how successive improvements in tools enhanced the lives and productivity of the farm families. Tours of the 19th-century mansion are given on weekends April–October. The formal gardens are a must-see with their azaleas, crepe myrtles, and boxwoods. This side of the James is most directly accessed via the Jamestown–Scotland Wharf Ferry, while the closest

bridge to the east is in Newport News and to the west is in Charles City County.

Shortly after turning into the park's main entrance, you'll see a sign for the campground on the right just across from the swimming pool. Chippokes was named for an American Indian chief who befriended early English settlers.

The park has two campground loops, with campground A's 30 wooded sites providing shade for tent campers and RVs up to 30 feet long. Campground B has sites that will accommodate RVs up to 50 feet long. All campsites have electric and water hookups, but tent campers will clearly prefer campground A.

The park has 3.5 miles of paved trails for hikers and bikers. Scheduled nature activities include guided fossil walks along the James River waterfront and canoe trips on the quiet streams that teem with both indigenous and migratory wildlife of the lower James River.

If you're looking to venture further afield and continue your colonial history lessons, head over to Scotland Wharf (about 5 miles away). From there, take the 15-minute ferry ride to Jamestown. Colonial Williamsburg is a scant 10 miles away on the Colonial Parkway, perhaps one of the most beautiful roads in America. Another 15 miles on the parkway will take you to the

## :: Ratings

BEAUTY: ★ ★ ★ ★
SITE PRIVACY: ★ ★ ★
SPACIOUSNESS: ★ ★ ★
QUIET: ★ ★ ★
SECURITY: ★ ★
CLEANLINESS: ★ ★ ★ ★ ★

## :: Key Information

| | |
|---|---|
| **ADDRESS:** 695 Chippokes Park Road, Surry, VA 23883 | **PARKING:** 1 vehicle in addition to camping unit at campsite; overflow parking at swimming pool |
| **OPERATED BY:** Virginia Department of Conservation and Recreation | **FEE:** Campground A $27 per night; campground B $30 per night |
| **CONTACT:** 757-294-3625; virginiastateparks.gov | **ELEVATION:** 100 feet |
| **OPEN:** March–first Monday in December | **RESTRICTIONS:** |
| **SITES:** 48 | ▦ **Pets:** On leash and not allowed in swimming areas or restrooms; $3 surcharge |
| **SITE AMENITIES:** Electricity, water, picnic table, lantern pole, fire ring, tent pad | ▦ **Fires:** In fire rings, stoves, or grills only |
| **ASSIGNMENT:** Your choice | ▦ **Alcohol:** Public drinking is prohibited |
| **REGISTRATION:** Call 800-933-PARK or visit reserveamerica.com. Site assignment on arrival | ▦ **Vehicles:** Up to 50 feet |
| **FACILITIES:** Swimming pool, cabin rental, flush toilets, hot showers, drink machines, pay phone | ▦ **Other:** Do not carve, chop, or damage any live trees; keep noise at a reasonable level; no boat launching at park; maximum stay is 14 days in a 30-day period |

Yorktown Battlefield, where the Revolutionary War ended. From the north side of the James River, those less interested in history and more intent on contemporary entertainment can head for the roller coasters of Busch Gardens or the water slides of Water Country USA.

Chippokes and I go back to the early 1970s, when, as an undergraduate at the College of William and Mary, I would venture across the James River and pedal around the quiet, rural backroads of Surry County. Surry seems to have changed very little in the intervening 40-some years, so road cycling along the county's little-traveled roads is still an enjoyable activity while visiting Chippokes.

In addition to cycling, paddlers will find much to enjoy in the area with a park located on the James River. Although Chippokes does not have its own boat launch, you'll find one of my favorite spots across the river. A mile or so down Jamestown Road heading toward Williamsburg is the Powhatan Creek

landing on the left side. I have kayaked here numerous times and enjoyed great birding, including all kinds of ducks, geese, herons, and bald eagles both on and above this waterway that wends its way past replicas of the three historic ships at Jamestown and into the James itself.

Equestrians will also find the 8.2-mile Chippokes Creek Equestrian Trail to be an enjoyable way to explore part of the park along a fairly easy gravel path that follows the edge of fields and connects the woodlands along the James River to the historic area and the length of Cedar Lane. The Equestrian Area also includes a corral and running water for horses.

An especially fun time to visit is in July, when the annual Pork, Pine, and Peanut Festival takes place at Chippokes, where you can sample some of the best pork and peanut dishes; enjoy down-home bluegrass, country, and gospel music; and admire the craftsmanship of more than 230 artisans.

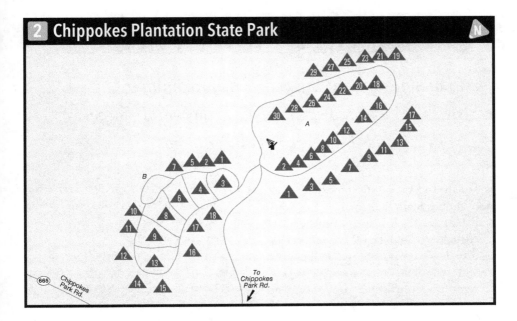

Campers should plan to spend at least a few days at Chippokes to get a complete picture of the natural and historic aspects of the park and surrounding Surry County. Bird-watchers, history buffs, and those who enjoy outdoor recreation will find a haven on the quiet side of the James River. Just be sure to bring ample insect repellent and an adventurous soul.

## :: Getting There

From Williamsburg, follow Jamestown Road (VA 31) south to the James River ferry dock. Cross the river and continue south on VA 31 to Surry. Turn left onto VA 10 at the town center, and then left onto VA 634.

Continue 4 miles to the park entrance. Park is also accessible via VA 10 coming west from Smithfield and east from Hopewell.

**GPS COORDINATES**   N37° 08.497 W76° 44.456

# 3

# First Landing State Park

*First Landing's greatest appeal is its proximity to the activities of Virginia Beach, billed as the world's largest resort beach and the largest city in Virginia.*

**Seashore State Park** (now called First Landing State Park) joined five other state parks as the first to be launched into the fledgling Virginia park system on June 15, 1936. It was renamed First Landing State Park in 1999, but Virginia traditions tend to remain, so you'll find many folks who still refer to it as Seashore State Park. While much is known about the role of Jamestown in the settlement of the New World, the park's current name reflects the lesser-known fact that the Virginia Company landed first at this site on the Chesapeake Bay on April 26, 1607, before proceeding to Jamestown on May 13. Among First Landing's current distinctions: It's the most visited park in Virginia's system, drawing more than 1 million visitors annually. First Landing's greatest appeal is its proximity to the activities of Virginia Beach, billed as the world's largest resort beach and the largest city in Virginia. For campers who crave solitude when pitching a tent, however, the park's popularity and location in

## :: Ratings

BEAUTY: ★ ★ ★
SITE PRIVACY: ★ ★ ★
SPACIOUSNESS: ★ ★ ★
QUIET: ★ ★
SECURITY: ★ ★
CLEANLINESS: ★ ★

a city of approximately 430,000 people can be its biggest detractors. However, rolling dunes and live oaks form effective buffers between many sites.

Shore Drive, also known as US 60, divides First Landing's campground from its trail system and day-use area, so traffic through the campground is limited to campers and their vehicles. Additionally, the beachfront swimming area is open only to overnight guests, so don't let the 1 million visitors discourage you from spending the night here. Two large loops fan out to the right and left of the campground entrance station for access to the 188 sites, which are separated by small sand dunes and trees. Tent campers are not allowed on the beachside sites, but it's just a short walk from most sites to the beach via convenient boardwalks across the dunes.

First Landing's 20 miles of trails can be accessed from the visitor center on the opposite side of US 60 from the campground. The 6-mile (point-to-point) Cape Henry Trail is extremely popular among bicyclists and stays busy, especially on weekends during the summer. Those out for a nice walk should keep that in mind and stick to the other 19 miles of trails that restrict bicycles. They range from the 0.3-mile Fox Run Trail to the 5-mile Long Creek Trail. Besides the usual coastal landscape that you might expect to find here where the

## :: Key Information

**ADDRESS:** 2500 Shore Drive, Virginia Beach, VA 23451-9645

**OPERATED BY:** Virginia Department of Conservation and Recreation

**CONTACT:** 757-412-2300; virginiastateparks.gov

**OPEN:** March–first Monday in December

**SITES:** 188

**SITE AMENITIES:** Picnic table, fire ring, lantern pole; electric/water hookups available on some sites

**ASSIGNMENT:** First come, first served

**REGISTRATION:** Call 800-933-PARK or visit reserveamerica.com; site assignment on arrival

**FACILITIES:** Chesapeake Bay beach access, boat launch, water, hot showers, laundry, camp store, pay phone

**PARKING:** 1 vehicle per site in addition to camping unit

**FEE:** Standard site $24 per night; $32 per night with electric/water hookups

**ELEVATION:** At sea level

**RESTRICTIONS:**
- **Pets:** On leash or in enclosed area; in swimming areas on leash with overnight guests only
- **Fires:** In fire rings, stoves, or grills only
- **Alcohol:** Prohibited
- **Vehicles:** Up to 34 feet
- **Other:** Do not damage any trees; bicycles only on park roads and the Cape Henry Trail; no motorized vehicles on trails; maximum stay is 14 days in a 30-day period; quiet hours 10 p.m.–6 a.m.

Atlantic Ocean meets the Chesapeake Bay, the park is the northernmost location on the East Coast where you can see both subtropical and temperate plants growing together. It was included in the National Register of Natural Landmarks in 1965. As you walk through sand dunes that reach as high as 75 feet, don't be surprised to see Spanish moss hanging from bald cypress, wild olive, live oak, and beech trees.

Described as the park's most popular trail, the 1.5-mile Bald Cypress Trail starts from the visitor center and loops along boardwalks through cypress swamps complete with resident pileated woodpeckers and turtles sunning themselves on logs. The Long Creek Trail starts at the main park, beginning on the park's main road, and winds through salt marshes past osprey nests, great blue herons, and egrets stalking their prey.

False Cape State Park, the least-visited state park in Virginia, is located just a few miles away in the community of Sandbridge. False Cape's ranking can be attributed to its limited access, which is restricted to bicycle, boat, and foot. Additionally, day users can ride the electric tram in the summer and the low-impact, beach-oriented "Terra Gator" in the winter. Campers must hike, bike, or boat the 6 miles to the primitive campsites, which reward them with a secluded night on this near-pristine barrier peninsula.

For some, camping at First Landing State Park is more an inexpensive way to stay in a bustling resort city than an opportunity to get away from their own particular rat race. However, others will access the park's sandy beaches along the Chesapeake Bay rather than fight the crowds along the oceanfront. First Landing's 188 campsites are as diverse as they are plentiful in terms

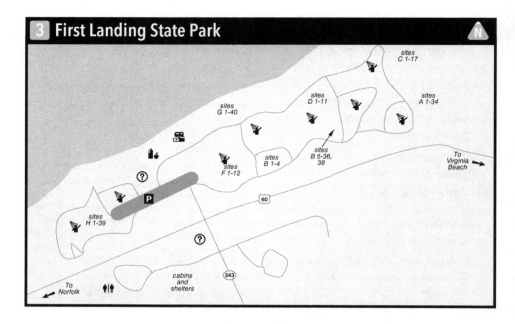

of the privacy, available hookups, and type of camping conveyance they accommodate. Tent campers will find many sites to their liking, but those looking for the optimum getaway experience will shun those backing up to the traffic noise of Shore Drive in favor of interior sites closer to the Chesapeake Bay.

Reservations are strongly recommended if you plan to stay here during the summer, as this is Virginia's most popular state park. If you plan to enjoy the pleasures and natural beauty that First Landing State Park has to offer, schedule your visit during the week or outside of the busy summer months.

## :: Getting There

From I-64, take Exit 282 heading north on US 13. After eight traffic lights, turn right onto US 60/Shore Drive, the last exit before the Chesapeake Bay Bridge Tunnel. Go 4.5 miles to the park's entrance.

**GPS COORDINATES**   N36° 55.117  W76° 03.151

# 4

# Kiptopeke State Park

*The drive across and under the bay coupled with the one-way toll is a small price to pay for the tranquility that you'll find on the Eastern Shore.*

**K**iptopeke **State** Park is located at the southern end of Virginia's Eastern Shore, just 3 miles from the Chesapeake Bay Bridge-Tunnel. Separated from the "mainland" of the Old Dominion by the 20-mile bridge-tunnel, the Eastern Shore is an entirely different world with a much slower pace than the one you left behind in Norfolk. The drive over and under the bay is a great way to begin your journey to the tranquility of the Eastern Shore. This 540-acre park offers 4,276 feet of beachfront for swimming, surf casting, or just a leisurely stroll while watching the sunset.

After leaving US 13 and entering Kiptopeke (which translates to "big water"), you'll find the campground on the right just a short distance up the park's main road. The campsites are arranged in rows and vary from full hookups to no hookups and from open field to dense pine woods. The campsites become more wooded with higher numbers: 1–94 are mostly open and include hookups for electricity, water, and sewer,

## :: Ratings

BEAUTY: ★ ★ ★ ★
SITE PRIVACY: ★ ★ ★
SPACIOUSNESS: ★ ★ ★
QUIET: ★ ★ ★ ★
SECURITY: ★ ★ ★
CLEANLINESS: ★ ★ ★ ★

while 95–141 are wooded tent sites without hookups. As you'd expect, this campground at just 25 feet above sea level is mostly flat, so there are options as to where to set up your tent on any given site. In choosing a temporary home site at Kiptopeke, however, keep in mind that woods can be both a plus and a minus when you're camping on the coast. They provide privacy from other campers, but the heavy growth of pines and underbrush also cuts off welcome breezes that can cool a sultry summer day and push pesky, six-legged critters right past your site. If you neglected to pack your tent, you can rent the Kiptopeke yurt. Other overnight accommodations at Kiptopeke State Park include five multibedroom lodges, rental RVs, and a bunkhouse. Boardwalks from the campground cross the sand dunes to reach the beach a short walk away.

Standing on the beach looking west across the Chesapeake, you'll spot stationary ships just offshore. These partially submerged concrete ships, sometimes called the Kiptopeke Navy, provided a harbor for the Virginia Ferry Corporation, which ran as many as 90 daily Chesapeake Bay crossings to Virginia Beach between 1933 and 1964 when the Chesapeake Bay Bridge-Tunnel was opened. Today these ships that were purchased in 1948 are habitats, their only passengers being birds and sea creatures. A Virginia saltwater fishing license is required

## :: Key Information

**ADDRESS:** 3540 Kiptopeke Drive, Cape Charles, VA 23310

**OPERATED BY:** Virginia Department of Conservation and Recreation

**CONTACT:** 757-331-2267; virginiastateparks.gov

**OPEN:** First weekend in March–first Monday in December

**SITES:** 141

**SITE AMENITIES:** Picnic table, fire ring, lantern pole

**ASSIGNMENT:** Campers can choose from available sites

**REGISTRATION:** Call 800-933-PARK or visit reserveamerica.com; site assignment on arrival

**FACILITIES:** Swimming in Chesapeake Bay, overnight lodge, yurt and RV rental, hot showers, pay phone, camp store

**PARKING:** 1 vehicle in addition to camping unit

**FEE:** $24 per night; $32 per night with electric/water hookups; $37 per night with electricity, water, and sewer

**ELEVATION:** 30 feet

**RESTRICTIONS:**

■ **Pets:** On leash or in enclosed area; not allowed on swimming beach; $3 per night

■ **Fires:** In fire rings, stoves, or grills only

■ **Alcohol:** Public drinking is prohibited

■ **Vehicles:** Up to 40 feet

■ **Other:** Do not damage trees; maximum of 6 people or 1 family per site; maximum stay is 14 days in a 30-day period; Feb. 15–April 30 campfires are allowed 4 p.m.–12 a.m. only

to fish from the shore, but none is needed when casting off the park's pier. The park also has its own boat launch with 4.5 feet depth at mean low water.

Bird-watchers flock to the area in October for the Eastern Shore Birding Festival to observe some of the more than 200,000 birds of prey and migratory birds that use this flyway. The park has been the site of bird-banding programs for population studies since 1963. Volunteers catch, examine, band, and release birds September–November. The hawk observatory platform and banding station are located on the opposite side of the park road from the campground. Park personnel conduct guided hikes, campfire programs, scavenger hunts, and other fun,

educational activities that are unique to this Eastern Shore locale.

Additional birding grounds can be found at the 1,200-acre Eastern Shore of Virginia National Wildlife Refuge, a short distance south on US 13. To fully experience the refuge, take a sea kayak tour offered by Southeast Expeditions (877-kayak-11) in nearby Cheriton. The massive Cherrystone Family Camping Resort is also in Cheriton. While it is geared toward RVs, its activities include minigolf, tennis courts, water balloon games, and an arcade, making it popular with kids. Additionally, Assateague Island National Seashore, 106 miles north, is famous among young ones for its wild ponies. The campground is on the Maryland side of the park.

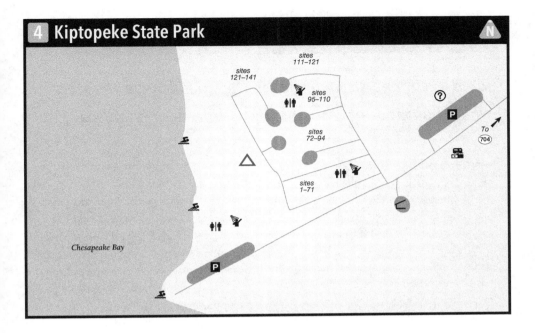

## :: Getting There

From Norfolk, cross the Chesapeake Bay Bridge-Tunnel on US 13. After 3 miles turn left onto VA 704, and continue until you reach the park entrance.

**GPS COORDINATES**   N37° 10.316  W75° 58.729

# 5

# Newport News Park

*Pitch a tent and sleep nestled in the woods under the stars while thousands of cars whiz by within earshot on I-64.*

The 8,000-acre Newport News Park, one of the largest municipal parks east of the Mississippi River, has shone brighter and brighter as development (and corresponding traffic) in the Hampton Roads area of Virginia has increased. Like many urban parks, it offers a vast array of activities for both campers and day users, including a lake for boating and fishing, an 18-hole disc golf course, an archery range, 30 miles of hiking trails, a family-oriented 5.3-mile bike path, and a 5-mile singletrack mountain bike trail.

Newport News Park is located between Newport News and Williamsburg along I-64, Jefferson Avenue, and Fort Eustis Boulevard. After pulling off Jefferson Avenue into the park, you'll stop at the camp store and office to register. Continuing along the park road, you'll see the six campground loops (A–F) on the right. The 188 campsites are nestled in the woods, where campers can pitch a tent and sleep under the stars while thousands of cars whiz by within earshot on I-64 and VA 143.

Loop E and its sites without electric hookups will probably look the most attractive to minimalist campers. If you'd like to camp along the reservoir's edge, make a beeline for one of the following: B35–38, 41, 42, 44, 46, 48, 50, 51, and 53. Sites F171, 172, 174, 175, 177, and 178 are also waterfront. All sites are flat, offer ample distance from other sites, and lie within a grove of mature hardwoods with some understory. Be sure to bring bug spray, as this is a low-lying area.

Camping at Newport News Park while sightseeing the regional attractions is a popular and economical alternative to high-priced hotels. The park itself, however, offers several recreational options within walking and biking distance. These include the archery range, two 18-hole golf courses at Deer Run, an 18-hole disc golf course, and a 30-acre aeromodel flying field. Nature programs suitable for children and adults occur regularly, in addition to the Children's Festival of Friends, the Newport News Fall Festival of Folklife, and the Celebration in Lights at Christmas, when 450,000 lights transform the park into a magical place.

The park's bike path is popular among both cyclists and joggers. Its flat, sandy surface offers the opportunity for some leisurely exercise. Those looking to expand their adventure past the park's boundaries can take the turn for Washington's Headquarters located between the 2- and 3-mile markers. Taking this detour provides access to the Colonial National Historical Park at

## :: Ratings

BEAUTY: ★ ★ ★
SITE PRIVACY: ★ ★ ★
SPACIOUSNESS: ★ ★ ★
QUIET: ★ ★ ★
SECURITY: ★ ★
CLEANLINESS: ★ ★ ★

## :: Key Information

**ADDRESS:** 13564 Jefferson Avenue, Newport News, VA 23603

**OPERATED BY:** City of Newport News Department of Parks

**CONTACT:** 757-888-3333; newport-news.va.us/parks

**OPEN:** Year-round

**SITES:** 188

**SITE AMENITIES:** Picnic table, fire ring, grill

**ASSIGNMENT:** Campers can choose from available sites

**REGISTRATION:** Call 800-203-8322 or on arrival

**FACILITIES:** Fishing, boating, archery range, 18-hole golf course, laundry room, camp store, hot showers, water, flush toilets, pay phones, drink machine

**PARKING:** 2 private vehicles per campsite

**FEE:** $28.50 per night; $30.50 per night with electric hookup; $31 per night with electric/water hookups

**ELEVATION:** 40 feet

**RESTRICTIONS:**

■ **Pets:** On leash only with proof of rabies vaccination

■ **Fires:** Must be attended; dead and down wood may be used for firewood

■ **Other:** Pitch tents within 25 feet of the pad with no more than 2 tents per site and only 1 camping vehicle per site; quiet hours 11 p.m.–8 a.m.; maximum length of stay is 21 days within a 30-day period April 1–Oct. 31

Yorktown, where the last battle of the Revolutionary War was fought in 1781.

Hikers can stretch their legs on 30 additional miles of trails, but bikers are restricted to the bike path and roads. Nature lovers should visit the trails located in the park's swampy area between the Deer Run Golf Course and the bike path just off the eastern edge of the Lee Hall Reservoir.

Johnboats, canoes, and paddleboats are available for rent should you want to fish for bass, pickerel, pike, or perch or just want to take a leisurely sojourn around the 650 acres of freshwater provided by the park's two reservoirs.

Stop by the Interpretive Center to get a better idea of the park's place in the past and present. The park features some three dozen species of mammals, more than 200 species of birds, Civil War earthworks, and a number of family events. Many other activities are available in the surrounding region. Those trying to stay in touch with Mother Nature will want to visit the nearby Virginia Living Museum with its live animal exhibits in natural habitats, planetarium, and 4,000-gallon ocean aquarium. Those interested in history can visit Colonial Williamsburg, while the roller coasters of Busch Gardens and waterslides of Water Country USA offer relief for kids and the young-at-heart. Information about area attractions is available from park headquarters and at the Tourist Information Center just east of the campsite office entrance on Jefferson Avenue.

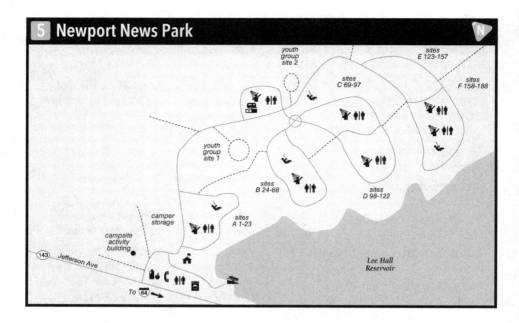

## :: Getting There

From I-64, take Exit 250B and follow the signs a short distance on Jefferson Avenue.
**GPS COORDINATES**   N37° 11.296  W76° 33.502

# 6

# Northwest River Park

*This land was once cultivated farmland, but shadier activities also went on here.*

**N**orthwest River Park's 763 acres lie on the coastal plain near the southern border of Virginia. Those coming for the day or to spend a few nights will find peace and quiet, with Indian Creek, Northwest River, and Smith Creek surrounding the park on three sides and a 29-acre lake meandering through the middle of it. Don't worry about arriving unprepared to enjoy the water because paddleboats and canoes are available for rent. You may also enjoy fishing in the stocked 6-acre freshwater lake for bass, bluegill, crappie, catfish, and trout. This land was once cultivated farmland, but shadier activities also went on here. More than 30 sites for making moonshine have been found on the property, including four in the area known as Moonshine Meadow. Alcoholic beverages are currently prohibited.

After entering the park from Indian Creek Road, you'll arrive at the six-sided camp store and office next to the lake and boat-rental area. Across the gravel road is the minigolf course. After registering, take the gravel road to the right to reach the campground. The campground consists of 66 sites set out on two loops among a grove of towering oaks. The area is flat and shaded with little vegetative barrier between sites. They are spacious, however, with substantial distances between sites. Of the 19 nonelectric tent sites, the most popular and private ones are 52, 53, 55, 58, 59, 61, 63, 65, 67, 68, and 70, which lie on the campground's outer edge. A backdrop of bamboo and hardwoods shields these sites but can also stifle breezes. This can be an important consideration when camping in low-lying and potentially buggy areas. Pack an ample supply of bug spray.

There are specific rules pertaining to the Equestrian Area, which is situated between the campground and the Indian Creek launch. This area provides for equestrian camping as well as those trails on which horseback riding is permitted.

Don't feel confined to the park's boundaries when looking for adventures on the water. From the confluence of Indian Creek and Northwest River at Otter Point, it's just a couple of miles to the North Carolina border. In addition to paddling through the lazy waters that surround the park, there are other activities for outdoorsy folk. The trails at Northwest River Park offer chances to view the swampy topography up close. Wood ducks and river otters live in this environment, as does marsh vegetation,

## :: Ratings

BEAUTY: ★ ★ ★
SITE PRIVACY: ★ ★ ★
SPACIOUSNESS: ★ ★ ★
QUIET: ★ ★ ★
SECURITY: ★ ★ ★
CLEANLINESS: ★ ★ ★ ★

## :: Key Information

**ADDRESS:** 1733 Indian Creek Road, Chesapeake, VA 23322

**OPERATED BY:** City of Chesapeake Parks and Recreation Department

**CONTACT:** 757-421-7151 or 757-421-3145; cityofchesapeake.net

**OPEN:** April 1–Nov. 30

**SITES:** 66

**SITE AMENITIES:** Picnic table, fire ring

**ASSIGNMENT:** By campground management

**REGISTRATION:** By reservation up to 90 days in advance or on arrival

**FACILITIES:** Fishing and paddling on Lake Lesa, camp store, pay phone, laundry room, vending machines, equestrian campground

**PARKING:** 2 vehicles per campsite

**FEE:** Standard tent site $21 per night; $26 per night with electric hookup

**ELEVATION:** Sea level

**RESTRICTIONS:**

■ **Pets:** Attended and on leash; clean up after pet

■ **Fires:** Attended on cooking pits only; no tree cutting

■ **Alcohol:** Prohibited

■ **Vehicles:** 2 per site

■ **Other:** No loud noise; quiet time 10 p.m.–7 a.m.; no firearms or other weapons; swimming prohibited; campsite water outlets not for vehicles, dishes, clothes, or bathing; no more than 14 consecutive nights

such as water tupelo, bald cypress, mistletoe, and Christmas fern. Trails range in length from the 0.75-mile Deer Island Trail to the 2.5-mile Indian Creek Trail. The Deer Island Trail is accessible near the campground entrance and near Shuttle Road, where several of the other trails also emerge. Along the Indian Creek Trail you'll find the arched hickory tree and the resurrection fern, which turns brown when dry and then green again when it rains. The 1.5-mile Molly Mitchell Trail, located on the northeastern corner of the park, was named in honor of former landowners who lived where the group picnic shelter now stands. The Scenic Slough provides a habitat for wood ducks, otters, squirrels, reptiles, and amphibians. The 1-mile Otter Point Trail can be found on the southern edge of Northwest River Park. Among the park's bald cypress trees, there is one towering specimen that has a large base and is thought to be several hundred years old.

Bikes are not allowed on the trails but are a comfortable way to get around the park's sandy roads. Should you bring your two-wheeler, be sure to pedal along the Shuttle Road out to the Southern Terminal. This grassy open area offers a great spot for a picnic, dropping a fishing line, or communing with nature at the confluence of Indian Creek, Smith Creek, and the Northwest River. A short, winding boardwalk trail loops around the fragrance garden for those who are visually impaired or just enjoy a sweet-smelling garden. It's located next to the camp store. All of the park's trails are clearly marked and impeccably maintained.

And turning your gaze skyward, you can learn about the heavens with the Back Bay Amateur Astronomers, who meet monthly in the evenings at the Equestrian Area.

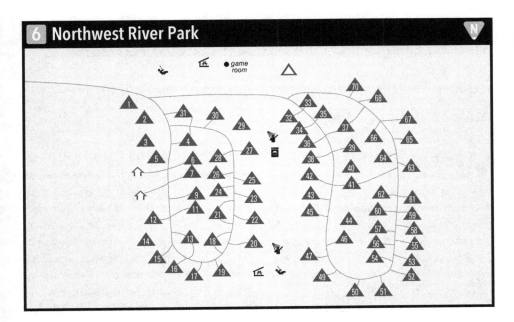

## :: Getting There

From I-64, take the Battlefield Boulevard exit (VA 168) heading south. Continue 15 miles and turn left onto Indian Creek Road. Go 4 miles to the campground entrance.

**GPS COORDINATES**   N36° 35.168  W76° 09.157

# 7

# Westmoreland State Park

*Explore Westmoreland March–November when its three campgrounds are open.*

**W**estmoreland State Park, located on Virginia's rural Northern Neck peninsula, is best known for its views of the Potomac from the Horsehead Cliffs. Additionally, the park is positioned between the birthplaces of both George Washington and Robert E. Lee, its campgrounds providing history buffs with an economical alternative to hotels.

The campgrounds are closed in the off-season, but the 1,299-acre park itself is open. Set aside the Horsehead Cliffs, and instead stroll the 7 miles of sandy paths crisscrossing the park to view the seasonal and abundant holly that stands out against the somber deciduous oak, hickory, and beech forest. Festooned with bright red berries set against shining green leaves, the holly branches sing of the season and fill the woods with cheer.

Established in 1936, Westmoreland was one of Virginia's first six state parks. Apart from the holiday season, it's best to explore Westmoreland March–November when its three campgrounds are open. After turning off VA 3 in the village of Baynesville onto VA 347, it's a mile to the park's contact station. Continuing, you'll arrive first at campground C, on the right, where the park road's two lanes divide around a wooded median. The first of these 40 sites alternate on either side of the campground road until a loop forms, housing sites 14–40. It's on this loop that campers desiring a little privacy will want to pitch their nylon getaway. Site 34 is particularly well secluded from the beaten path. It is also adjacent to the 2.5-mile Turkey Neck Trail, which loops around the eastern section of the park.

The dual lanes of the 2-mile park road rejoin after a short distance; look for campground B on the left. Just before the entrance is the trailhead for the half-mile Rock Spring Pond Trail, which joins the 1.3-mile Laurel Point Trail to loop around to the beachfront on the Potomac River. Campground B has 51 sites spread out along interconnected looping campground roads, while thick plantings of holly provide a colorful understory beneath mature hardwoods. Approximately two-thirds of the sites offer electric and water hookups, but these sites are more conducive to pop-up campers than to recreational vehicles. Especially enticing are sites 33–45 and 46–56, which are situated along their own smaller loops. Campground A is located between the park's visitor center and the camp store on the right side of the park road, but these 38 sites are designed to accommodate large RVs as well as six small cabins.

## :: Ratings

BEAUTY: ★ ★ ★ ★
SITE PRIVACY: ★ ★ ★
SPACIOUSNESS: ★ ★ ★
QUIET: ★ ★ ★
SECURITY: ★ ★ ★
CLEANLINESS: ★ ★ ★ ★

## :: Key Information

**ADDRESS:** 1650 State Park Road, Montross, VA 22520

**OPERATED BY:** Virginia Department of Conservation and Recreation

**CONTACT:** 804-493-8821; virginiastateparks.gov

**OPEN:** March–first Monday in December

**SITES:** 129

**SITE AMENITIES:** Picnic table and fire grill

**ASSIGNMENT:** First come, first served

**REGISTRATION:** Call 800-933-PARK or visit reserveamerica.com; site assignment on arrival

**FACILITIES:** Rental cabins, boat launch, swimming pool, flush toilets, hot showers, laundry, restaurant, camp store

**PARKING:** At campsites, trailheads, and day-use area

**FEE:** Standard tent site $20 per night; $27 per night with electric/water hookups

**ELEVATION:** 160 feet

**RESTRICTIONS:**

■ **Pets:** Must be kept in an enclosed area or on a leash

■ **Fires:** In camp stoves and fire rings only

■ **Alcohol:** Public use is prohibited

■ **Vehicles:** Up to 40 feet

■ **Other:** Swimming not allowed from shoreline, but pool free to campers; maximum stay is 14 days in a 30-day period

Westmoreland's main road curves past the rental cabin areas before ending at the park's boat landing and swimming pool on the Potomac River beachfront. Anglers can fish for striped bass, spot, and bluefish from the pier or shore without a license, while fishing from a boat into the Potomac requires a Virginia or Maryland saltwater license. Seven hiking trails, including the new 0.4-mile Beach Trail, wind through the park, with Turkey Neck and Laurel Point being the longest. The others are all less than a mile and connect to the Turkey Neck and Laurel Point Trails. None of the trails are open to equestrians or bicyclists.

In addition to fishing, boating, and hiking on the park's maze of easy trails, Westmoreland features a variety of outdoor activities, including the old-fashioned Market Day, an orienteering meet sponsored by the Quantico Orienteering Club, and an outdoor photography workshop. And what better way to see the famed 150-foot Horsehead Cliffs up close than by taking one of the Kayak Below the Cliffs outings. Kids of all ages will enjoy hunting for sharks' teeth dating from nearly 23 million years ago at the base of the cliffs.

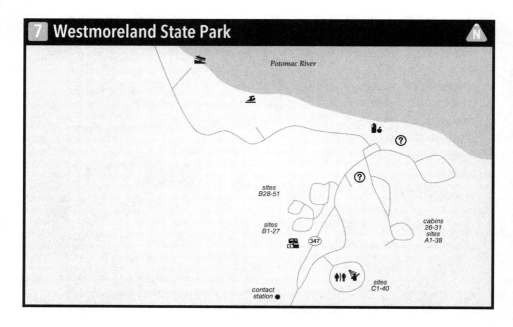

## :: Getting There

From I-95, take VA 3 at Fredericksburg, and drive 40 miles to the town of Baynesville. Turn left onto VA 347 to enter the park.

**GPS COORDINATES**   N38° 10.104  W76° 52.099

# The
# Piedmont

# 8

# Bear Creek Lake State Park

*Visitors can choose from an array of outdoor activities, including sunbathing, swimming, and practicing archery on the park's range.*

**B**ear Creek Lake State Park is a small park located near Richmond in Central Virginia's Cumberland State Forest. It features a variety of outdoor and water activities to keep both vacationers and urban refugees happy. The park's three campgrounds, designated A, B, and C, are nestled in the shade of mature towering sweet gum, oak, and tulip polar trees. There are 12 sites designated as tents only.

Campground A sits on a hillside overlooking 40-acre Bear Creek Lake just behind the camp office. The campground host's site is adjacent to the picnic shelter at site A14. The sites are fairly close together. If given a choice, try to snag sites 8, 9, 10, or 11, as they hug the lake. The small loop encompassing sites A4–12 has no hookups and is well suited to self-sufficient tent campers.

Campground B, with electric and water hookups, is the busiest of the three. It is located across the road from the camp office and features 20 sites on a single loop under a roof of hardwoods. The sites are close together, and the loop lacks a bathhouse.

Camping is popular in campground C. The single campsite loop is flat and has its own bathhouse. Campground C contains 11 sites, with sites 8 and 10 being the most private. The quarter-mile Running Cedar Trail is just across the road and provides access to the Lakeside Trail and swimming beach.

Over the past couple of years, Virginia's state park system has been busy adding lodgings to parks that did not have them. Be sure to check out this park's array of camping cabins, two- and three-bedroom cabins, and multibedroom lodges if you don't feel like roughing it.

Bear Creek Lake State Park's archery range is an enjoyable activity at the lake. Ten bale targets bearing faces of assorted big game—such as deer, bear, and turkey—are set against natural backdrops. Shooting stations are designated by color to allow easier, more consistent scoring. The range is open year-round, although closing times are dictated by light conditions and safety. Archers must bring their own gear.

Visitors can choose from an array of other outdoor activities, including sunbathing or swimming on the sandy beach. Anglers can fish throughout the year for largemouth bass, crappie, bream, and channel catfish. Other area lakes, including

## :: Ratings

BEAUTY: ★ ★ ★ ★
SITE PRIVACY: ★ ★
SPACIOUSNESS: ★ ★ ★
QUIET: ★ ★
SECURITY: ★ ★ ★
CLEANLINESS: ★ ★ ★ ★

## :: Key Information

**ADDRESS:** 22 Bear Creek Lake Road, Cumberland, VA 23040

**OPERATED BY:** Virginia Department of Conservation and Recreation

**CONTACT:** 804-492-4410; virginiastateparks.gov

**OPEN:** March 1- first Monday in December

**SITES:** 49

**SITE AMENITIES:** Picnic table, fire grill

**ASSIGNMENT:** Your choice

**REGISTRATION:** Call 800-933-PARK or visit reserveamerica.com; site assignment on arrival

**FACILITIES:** Cabin and lodge rental, lake swimming, fishing, boating, laundry sinks, pay phone, hot showers

**PARKING:** 1 vehicle in addition to camping unit allowed at site; overflow at office

**FEE:** Standard tent site $20 per night; $27 per night with electric/water hookups

**ELEVATION:** 270 feet

**RESTRICTIONS:**
- **Pets:** $5 per night; must be leashed
- **Fires:** In grills, camp stoves, or designated fire rings only
- **Alcohol:** Prohibited
- **Vehicles:** Up to 35 feet
- **Other:** Do not damage trees; no motorized vehicles on trails; scooters, skateboards, and in-line skates prohibited; maximum stay is 14 days in a 30-day period; quiet hours 11 p.m.–7 a.m.

Winston Lake, Arrowhead Lake, Oakhill Lake, and Bonbrook Lake, also provide fishing opportunities. A Virginia fishing license is required for those age 16 and older.

Paddleboats and canoes are available for rent during the summer. Both are available for trips around the lake, or check out one of the in-season family canoe tours.

There are a number of trails, both within the 326-acre park and in the surrounding 16,233-acre Cumberland State Forest. Some of the trails within the park are wheelchair accessible. The 1.5-mile (point-to-point) orange-blazed Lakeside Trail and the 3-mile white-blazed Lost Barr Trail hug opposite sides of the lake. The Lakeside Trail stretches from campground A past the lakeside picnic area and beach before connecting with Pine Knob Trail and Lost Barr Trail. Shorter walks in the park include the blue-blazed Running Cedar Trail, the 0.4-mile yellow-blazed Quail Ridge Trail, and quarter-mile gray-blazed Channel Cat Trail.

Hikers, equestrians, and mountain bikers looking for a longer jaunt can choose from either the blue-blazed 14-mile Cumberland Multi-Use Loop Trail or the 16-mile (point-to-point) Willis River Trail (bring your own horse). The Cumberland Multi-Use Loop Trail is fairly flat, with the exception of a few sections. Parking is located next to the Meeting Hall. Although it's a linear rather than a loop trail, all points of the Willis River Trail are within 10 miles of Bear Creek Lake State Park and can be accessed from intersections with county and state forest roads.

Between Memorial Day and Labor Day, Bear Creek Lake State Park also offers campfire talks and sing-alongs, night hikes, nature walks, junior ranger programs, and archery.

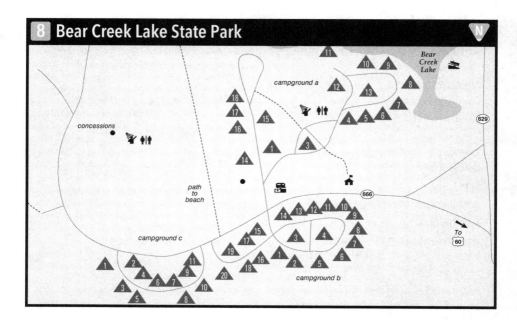

## :: Getting There

From US 60 east of Cumberland, go west on VA 622 and then south on VA 629 to the park entrance.

**GPS COORDINATES**   N37° 31.973  W78° 16.465

# 9

# Fairy Stone State Park

*The campground lies on one of the many hilltops here in the foothills of the Blue Ridge Mountains.*

**L**egend has it that a long time ago, fairies inhabited the foothills of the Blue Ridge Mountains in this section of Virginia near the North Carolina border. One day their play was interrupted by an elfin messenger who'd come from a distant city to bring news about the death of Christ. The fairies' grief was tremendous, and as their tears touched the earth, they formed beautiful crosses that symbolized the crucifixion. Although the fairies disappeared, these stone crosses remained and can still be found here today. Wearers of these fairy crosses long believed that they warded off witchcraft, sickness, accidents, and disaster. You may not put much stock in the myth, but there is no place in the world that offers either the quantity or the quality of shape of the brown staurolite crosses you find at Fairy Stone State Park.

The recommended spot for finding these unique stones can be found by heading east on VA 57 toward Bassett. After about 2.5 miles you'll notice the Fairy Stone Pitstop on the left. A sign identifies the park-owned property and streambed where the crosses can be collected for personal use. My then-13-year-old son, Chris, and I wandered along looking for these staurolite crosses with limited success. He half-expected the crystals to jump off the ground and into his hands, while I merely hoped that would be the case. The best time to go hunting is after a rain, but I was still able to find several examples during a dry spell. You're more likely to find the crystals still embedded in bits of schist, which is more easily weathered away, so patience and a good eye are essential. The judicious use of a file will bring out one of several shapes in which they form. Should you come up empty-handed, however, the Fairy Stone Pitstop offers a good selection at reasonable prices.

Fairy Stone was one of the six original parks in Virginia's park system in 1936. Its 4,639 acres made it the largest then, and it is still one of the largest today. After passing the 168-acre Fairy Stone Lake and beachfront on the left, you'll arrive at the contact station and the park office to the left of it. Straight ahead is the visitor center, where you'll want to stop to see the extensive collection of fairy stones, as well as information about the local history and plant and animal life. Bear right at the visitor center and continue a short distance up the road to the campground entrance on the left.

The campground lies on one of many hilltops in the foothills of the Blue Ridge

## :: Ratings

BEAUTY: ★ ★ ★
SITE PRIVACY: ★ ★
SPACIOUSNESS: ★ ★
QUIET: ★ ★ ★
SECURITY: ★ ★ ★
CLEANLINESS: ★ ★ ★

## :: Key Information

**ADDRESS:** 967 Fairystone Lake Drive, Stuart, VA 24171

**OPERATED BY:** Virginia Department of Conservation and Recreation

**CONTACT:** 276-930-2424; virginiastateparks.gov

**OPEN:** March 1–first Monday in December

**SITES:** 51

**SITE AMENITIES:** Picnic table, fire grill, electric/water hookups

**ASSIGNMENT:** First come, first served

**REGISTRATION:** Call 800-933-PARK or visit reserveamerica.com; site assignment on arrival

**FACILITIES:** Cabin and lodge rental; lake swimming, boating, and fishing; equestrian campground; flush toilets; hot showers; pay phone; drink machines (by swimming beach)

**PARKING:** 1 vehicle in addition to camping unit; additional parking a half mile away

**FEE:** $27 per night; includes electric/water hookups

**ELEVATION:** 1,240 feet

**RESTRICTIONS:**
■ **Pets:** On leash and attended; additional fee charged per night
■ **Fires:** In camp stoves and fire rings only
■ **Alcohol:** Public use prohibited
■ **Vehicles:** Up to 30 feet
■ **Other:** No cutting or marring of vegetation; maximum stay is 14 days in a 30-day period

Mountains. The 51 sites, all with electric and water hookups, enjoy the shade of a pine grove dotted with scattered oaks. Most of the campsites have sand tent pads, with the exception of several pull-throughs. The single loop is located in the center of the park off local roads. A dense barrier of pines and hardwoods surrounds the campground. Thick stands of wild rhododendron grow throughout the park; an especially large one is across from the picnic area leading up to the campground.

Fairy Stone State Park features several hiking trails that range in length and degree of challenge, from the 0.9-mile Beach Trail, which leads from site 28 to the lake and beach, to the orange-blazed Little Mountain Falls Trail. This 4.2-mile trail is accessible just across the road from the campground via the gated 2.1-mile Mountain View Hiking and Bicycle Trail. If you plan to hike, pick up one of the park's Stuart's Knob and Little Mountain Trail Systems Guides.

Besides the fairy stones themselves, the 168-acre Fairy Stone Lake is the centerpiece of this park. It offers swimming in the summer, as well as boating (self-propelled and electric motors only) and fishing for panfish and largemouth bass. Hardcore anglers and those with motorboats may want to leave the park and drive 30 minutes to reach the 2,880-acre Philpott Reservoir for some serious bass and walleye fishing.

There is a 10-site equestrian camp that will accommodate vehicles up to 50 feet. All of these sites have electric and water hookups and are pull-through. It also includes 10 covered stalls, which users are encouraged to maintain. Fairy Stone State Park's lodging options also include 25 cabins of varied sizes and a six-bedroom lodge that can be rented.

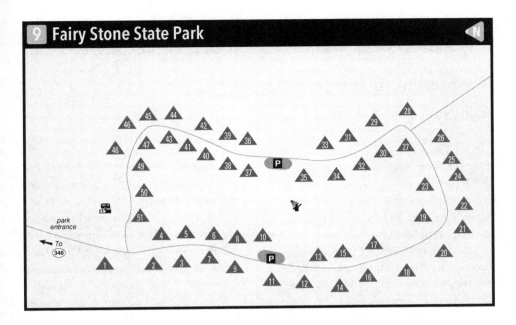

Over the past couple of years, Virginia's state park system has been busy adding lodgings to parks that did not have them. While it may seem like blasphemy to inveterate tent campers, I have learned that age (and a bad back) is oft accompanied by an appreciation for indoor plumbing, a proper bed, and a hard roof, underneath which rain can actually be enjoyed. Be sure to check out this park's array of camping cabins, two- and three-bedroom cabins, and multibedroom lodges.

## :: Getting There

From I-81 near Roanoke, take I-581 to US 220. Follow this to Bassett Forks, and turn right onto VA 57. Turn right onto VA 346, and continue until you reach the park's entrance.
**GPS COORDINATES** N36° 47.598 W80° 06.478

# 10

# Holliday Lake State Park

## The backdrop of mature hardwoods lends a woodsy feel to the area.

**A**mateur editors should take note that this park is named for the Holliday family farm, the remnants of which lie at the bottom of the lake, hence the unusual spelling. That bit of concern aside, feel free to enjoy the facilities that the 250-acre park has to offer. The campground is located to the right of the park road just after passing the contact station. It sits on the side of a hill, but fear not: The 30 sites are level and spacious, allowing ample room to pitch your tent. The backdrop of mature hardwoods lends a woodsy feel to the area, but the sites themselves are fairly open. As with most Virginia state parks, summer is a busy time here at Holliday Lake State Park, and reservations are highly recommended.

The park land and surrounding landscape were cleared for farming in the 1800s. However, the Federal Resettlement Administration began buying local tracts to return it to hardwood forest. The lake itself was constructed under the Works Progress Administration and completed in 1938. All the work was done by hand, with the assistance of mules and dynamite. The Commonwealth of Virginia took over managing what was then a day-use recreational area, and Holliday Lake became a state park in 1972 with the addition of campgrounds.

After passing the contact station, you'll quickly see the Laurel Ridge Campground on the right. These six sites are designated as RV sites and will accommodate vehicles up to 38 feet long. A little farther down the road (and closer to the sand beach) is the 30-site Redbud Campground, which tent campers will find much more to their liking. Tent pads have a fine gravel surface, and the three loops offer a camping experience with varying degrees of privacy. Sites 13, 14, and 15 are the most private, but they can accommodate tent campers as well as small trailers up to 22 feet long.

The short Saunders Creek Trail connects the campground and lakefront area. Here you'll find picnic shelters, a boat launch, and a swimming beach. Whether you want to fish the 150-acre lake for bass, crappie, or bluegill, you'll want to bring a boat (only electric motors can be used) or rent one to do some aquatic exploration. A Virginia fishing license is required to fish at Holliday Lake. The sandy beachfront swimming area offers a great way to cool off during the summer's heat, or have lunch alfresco in the shady, lakefront picnic area.

Besides swimming, fishing, and boating, another attraction here is the trailhead

## :: Ratings

BEAUTY: ★ ★ ★ ★
SITE PRIVACY: ★ ★
SPACIOUSNESS: ★ ★ ★ ★
QUIET: ★ ★
SECURITY: ★ ★ ★
CLEANLINESS: ★ ★ ★ ★

# :: Key Information

| | |
|---|---|
| **ADDRESS:** Route 2, Box 622, Appomattox, VA 24522 | **PARKING:** 1 vehicle in addition to camping unit allowed at site |
| **OPERATED BY:** Virginia Department of Conservation and Recreation | **FEE:** $27 per night with electric/water hookups |
| **CONTACT:** 434-248-6308; virginiastateparks.gov | **ELEVATION:** 470 feet |
| **OPEN:** March 1–first Monday in December | **RESTRICTIONS:** |
| **SITES:** 36 | ▪ **Pets:** Must be on short leash or enclosed; additional fee charged |
| **SITE AMENITIES:** Water, electricity, picnic table, fire grill, lantern pole | ▪ **Fires:** In fireplaces, fire rings, and camp stoves only |
| **ASSIGNMENT:** Upon arrival | ▪ **Alcohol:** Public use or display is prohibited |
| **REGISTRATION:** Call 800-933-PARK or visit reserveamerica.com; site assignment on arrival | ▪ **Vehicles:** Up to 38 feet |
| **FACILITIES:** Lake swimming, fishing, boating, playground, camp store, flush toilets, hot showers | ▪ **Other:** Maximum stay is 14 days in a 30-day period; maximum 6 people or a single family per site |

for the 12-mile Carter Taylor Loop Trail, which starts inside the park across from the campground. After quickly leaving the park and entering the surrounding 19,535-acre Appomattox-Buckingham State Forest, it utilizes state forest and state roads as well as the occasional stretch of singletrack. Pick up a Carter Taylor Loop Trail brochure, which shows the route of the multiuse trail open to hikers, bicyclists, and equestrians.

There are also shorter trails within the park's boundaries, including the 0.75-mile Dogwood Ridge Trail and the 5-mile Lakeshore Nature Trail. The Appomattox-Buckingham State Forest is Virginia's largest, with a considerable network of woods roads that are open to hikers, bikers, and equestrians. Those venturing out into the state forest should get a Virginia Forest Service map to stay oriented on the Carter Taylor as well as for assistance in developing additional

routes through the rolling countryside. Holliday Lake also features the unique Sunfish Aquatic Trail, a self-guided adventure that requires a boat to navigate.

Civil War buffs will not want to miss the opportunity to visit the Appomattox Court House National Historic Park, where Confederate General Robert E. Lee surrendered to Union General Ulysses S. Grant to end the Civil War, also known here in Virginia as the War of Northern Aggression. Be sure to visit the newly opened Museum of the Confederacy in Appomattox to see original artifacts and documents as well as audio and interactive displays that lead the visitor from the outbreak of war to the surrender of General Lee and his army at Appomattox. The exhibit continues into the years of reconstruction immediately after the war and beyond.

Lee's Army of Northern Virginia, weary and tattered, passed approximately 1.5 miles

## 10 Holliday Lake State Park

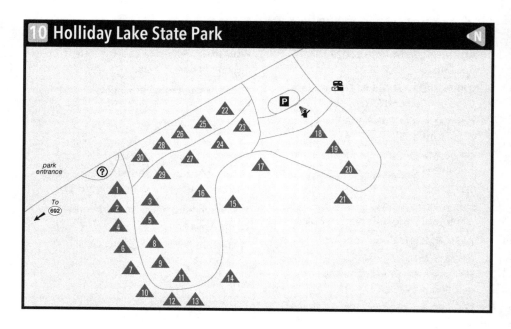

from the current park site en route to the final battles of the war. The park encompasses some 1,800 acres of rolling hills, with self-guided walking tours on the 6-mile History Trail, audiovisual programs, and various other interpretive programs presented by park personnel. The park's visitor center is located in the reconstructed courthouse on VA 24, just 2 miles northeast of the town of Appomattox.

## :: Getting There

From US 460, turn onto VA 24 in the town of Appomattox. After 8 miles, turn right onto VA 626 and follow it 3.4 miles. Turn left onto VA 640, and then right onto VA 692. Continue 2.5 miles to the park's entrance.

**GPS COORDINATES**   N37° 23.980 W78° 38.459

# 11

# James River State Park

*There is no privacy or undergrowth between riverfront sites, so campers must view their neighbors; however, the views of the river can't be beat.*

**James River State Park's** 1,500 acres are situated on 3 miles along Virginia's historic James River, so anglers, kayakers, canoeists, and tubers will have a ball here, especially during the sultry summer months. While James River access is a major draw, the park also features three fishing ponds, picnic areas, and 15 miles of trails for hikers, bikers, and equestrians.

There is an array of camping and lodging options to be found here. These include 20 primitive campsites (13 along the James and 7 at Branch Pond), 31 sites with electric and water hookups at Red Oak Campground, and a combination of 5 primitive and 5 full-hookup sites for equestrians, including 20 covered horse stalls.

Twenty-two sites sit near the James River at the canoe landing, with sites 1–14 being the closest. RVs up to 30 feet can be accommodated at some sites, including 9 riverfront drive-in sites, but there are several shaded tents-only sites along the river, just down a soft grassy bank. Campers must carry their gear approximately 40 feet from gravel parking spots to assigned tent sites. There is no privacy or undergrowth between sites, so campers must view their neighbors; however, the views of the river can't be beat. There are five primitive horse-camping sites and six stalls across the meadow from the canoe-landing sites.

The riverside campground is the star camping attraction at James River State Park, as it allows campers to launch canoes from their front yards at Dixon Landing. Nearby Branch Pond Campground is located in an idyllic, secluded forest. Campers searching for scenic privacy or lake fishing should set up in one of Branch Pond's seven wooded sites. A central parking area with a firewood stand is at the entrance to the campground, near three accessible sites and vault toilets. Large vans and SUVs should consider parking here, as the gravel road to the remaining sites is narrow with a tight turning radius. The sites have no hookups, and the three farthest sites are secluded enough that campers will think they are alone in the forest. Site 4 is desirably located on the lake, but the small public deck nearby may mean less privacy if the campground gets full. The decklike pier is covered and features picnic tables and a stone fireplace.

## :: Ratings

BEAUTY: ★ ★ ★ ★
SITE PRIVACY: ★ ★
SPACIOUSNESS: ★ ★ ★ ★
QUIET: ★ ★ ★
SECURITY: ★ ★
CLEANLINESS: ★ ★ ★

## :: Key Information

**ADDRESS:** 104 Green Hill Drive, Gladstone, VA 24553

**OPERATED BY:** Virginia Department of Conservation and Recreation

**CONTACT:** 434-933-4355; virginiastateparks.gov

**OPEN:** Primitive sites open year-round

**SITES:** 20 primitive; 31 with water and electricity; 10 equestrian sites with water and electricity

**SITE AMENITIES:** Picnic table, fire grill

**ASSIGNMENT:** Upon arrival

**REGISTRATION:** Call 800-933-PARK or visit reserveamerica.com; site assignment on arrival

**FACILITIES:** Equestrian campground, cabin rentals, vault toilets, and canoe landing for primitive sites; water,

restrooms at day-use area; modern bathhouse at Red Oak Campground

**PARKING:** 2 vehicles in addition to camping unit at site

**FEE:** Primitive sites $13 per night; Red Oak Campground $27 per night with electric/water hookups

**ELEVATION:** 450 feet

**RESTRICTIONS:**
- **Pets:** Must be on short leash or enclosed; $5 per night
- **Fires:** In camp stoves and fire rings only
- **Alcohol:** Prohibited
- **Vehicles:** Up to 30 feet
- **Other:** Maximum stay is 14 days in a 30-day period; maximum 6 people per site; dead wood may be collected

Outdoor Adventures is located at the canoe landing and offers a host of invaluable services, including sales and rental of various camping and paddling supplies. You need not leave the property to find fishing tackle, night crawlers, camp fuel, and lantern mantles. They also offer shuttle services, which river paddlers know make time on the water a lot more fun, especially when there is a decent current.

James River State Park has some 15 miles of multiuse trails, ranging in length from the 0.7-mile Dixon Trail to the 3.5-mile Cabell Trail. At the northern end of the park, the trails wind through pine forests. In the midsection, the park is rolling meadow, and toward the water, the terrain changes to diverse wetlands. Some of the trails are wheelchair accessible. There is no swimming in the park, but guided canoe floats, wagon rides, and campfire programs

are available in the summer. Horses are not available for rent, but bicycles can be rented at the park office May–September.

Aside from the nonpotable lakes and river, there is no running water in the primitive campgrounds, so campers should bring a large container and use it to carry water to their sites from the day-use areas. The word has gotten out about James River State Park, so online reservations at reserveamerica.com are a must. On the plus side, booking ahead means that sites are assigned ahead of time as well. Campers can request specific sites or adjacent sites, and the staff will try to accommodate them when they arrive at the park.

Over the past couple of years, Virginia's state park system has been busy adding lodgings to those parks that did not have them. While it may seem like blasphemy to inveterate tent campers, I have learned that

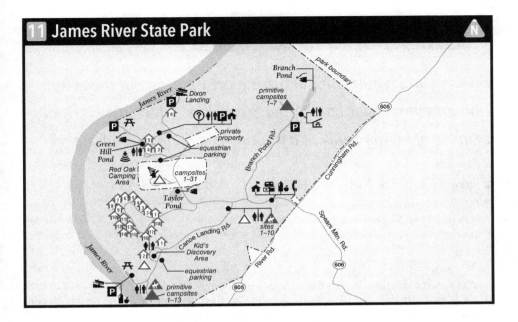

## 11 James River State Park

age (and a bad back) is oft accompanied by an appreciation for indoor plumbing, a proper bed, and a hard roof, underneath which rain can actually be enjoyed. Be sure to check out this park's array of camping cabins, two- and three-bedroom cabins, and multibedroom lodges.

## :: Getting There

From US 60 near Amherst, head north on VA 605 at the James River Bridge. Travel 7 miles, and then turn left onto VA 606.

**GPS COORDINATES**   N37° 37.424 W78° 47.977

# 12

# Lake Anna State Park

*Boating and fishing on Lake Anna are only part of the attraction for campers at Lake Anna State Park, which also includes 15 miles of hiking trails and a sandy beach for swimming.*

**L**ake Anna State Park provides many recreational opportunities, including access to one of Virginia's largest and most desirable lakes for motorboating and fishing. Largemouth bass, striped bass, and crappie are just a few of the fish that draw both amateur and professional anglers throughout the year. The park provides access to 10 miles of the lake's 200 miles of shoreline and the cold-water side of the 13,000-acre lake. Visitors should be aware that Dominion Power's North Anna Nuclear Power Station sits along the shoreline and uses the cold water from the public side of the lake to cool its system while depositing its warm effluent water into the private side of the lake. This power plant went into production in 1987. The park itself was previously known as Gold Hill and was the site of the Goodwin Gold Mine, where the precious metal was first found in 1829. It was continuously mined through the 1880s. The man-made lake was created in 1971, and work began the following year to develop Lake Anna State Park. It finally opened in 1983.

## :: Ratings

> BEAUTY: ★ ★ ★
> SITE PRIVACY: ★ ★
> SPACIOUSNESS: ★ ★ ★
> QUIET: ★ ★
> SECURITY: ★ ★
> CLEANLINESS: ★

The park has its own boat ramp, which is suitable for motorboats as well as canoes and kayaks. The adjacent parking lots are sized for vehicles with trailers and offer a large, shaded picnic area. Boating and fishing on Lake Anna are only part of the attraction for campers at the park, which also includes 15 miles of hiking trails and a sand beach for swimming at lake's edge. Twelve miles of trail are designated as multiuse, so plan to share those with mountain bikers and equestrians. Should you want to drown a few worms but not have a boat, fear not because there is a 2-acre fishing pond located next to the park's modern visitor center that is excellent for children and others with mobility impairment. Like other Virginia State Parks, staff and volunteers offer a number of special instructional adventure programs both on land and on water. These include Geocaching, Birding by the Beach, Paddle to the Meadow, Ware Creek Canoe Trip, Panning for Gold, and Night Hike. Check with park personnel at check-in to see what programs are being conducted and may be of interest.

Good-sized but open campsites are situated on two loops, with those with electric/water hookups interspersed throughout. One loop includes sites 1–17, while 18–46 lie along the second loop. Lake Anna State Park also features six camp cabins.

## :: Key Information

**ADDRESS:** 6800 Lawyers Road, Spotsylvania, VA 22551-9645

**OPERATED BY:** Virginia Department of Conservation and Recreation

**CONTACT:** 540-854-5503; dcr.virginia.gov

**OPEN:** March 1–early December

**SITES:** 46

**SITE AMENITIES:** Picnic table, fire ring, lantern pole; 23 sites include electric/water hookups

**ASSIGNMENT:** First come, first served

**REGISTRATION:** Call 800-933-PARK, visit reserveamerica.com, or on arrival; reservations highly recommended

**FACILITIES:** Water, hot showers, laundry, camp store, pay phone

**PARKING:** 1 vehicle per site in addition to camping unit

**FEE:** $24–$32 per night

**ELEVATION:** 280 feet

**RESTRICTIONS:**

■ **Pets:** On leash or in enclosed area; in swimming areas on leash with overnight guests only

■ **Fires:** In fire rings, stoves, or grills only

■ **Alcohol:** Prohibited

■ **Vehicles:** Up to 34 feet

■ **Other:** Do not damage any trees; bicycles only on park roads and the Cape Henry Trail; no motorized vehicles on trails; maximum stay is 14 days in a 30-day period; quiet hours 10 p.m.–6 a.m.

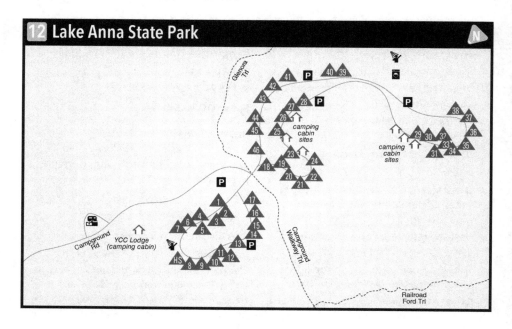

## :: Getting There

From I-64, take Exit 159 at Gum Springs. Take US 522 north 11 miles until you reach the village of Cuckoo. Stay on US 522 until you reach Mineral. Turn right at the traffic light, crossing railroad tracks. Take an immediate left onto US 522 north, and stay on the road 6 miles to the intersection just before Dickinson's Store. Take a right there onto VA 208 (New Bridge Road) and travel 8 miles. You'll cross a bridge. When you get to VA 601 (Lawyers Road), turn left and go 3 miles. The park sign will be on your left.

**GPS COORDINATES**   N38° 06.604  W77° 49.555

# 13

# Occoneechee State Park

*Park designers creatively arranged the tent-camping area to maximize privacy and excellent waterfront vistas.*

**The main** attraction at Occoneechee State Park is the 48,000-acre John H. Kerr Reservoir, also known as Buggs Island Lake. It is Virginia's largest lake. The park hugs the shoreline in the shadow of the Virginia–North Carolina boundary. Boaters and anglers alike flock to this lake, which is regarded highly for the quantity and size of its largemouth bass, bluegill, crappie, and perch. Canoe, kayak, and paddleboat rentals are available on summer weekends Memorial Day–Labor Day.

Occoneechee State Park is named for an American Indian tribe that inhabited a nearby island on the Roanoke River from 1250 until the late 1600s. The Occoneechee were friendly, entrepreneurial traders, but they were massacred by Virginia Councilman Nathaniel Bacon and a group of men from Henrico County during a power struggle with the government known as Bacon's Rebellion. To their credit, Governor Berkeley and the colonial British government rebuked Bacon for his actions. Descendants of the Occoneechee celebrate their ancestors every May at the park with the Native American Heritage Festival and Powwow. Those interested in more information about the American Indian presence should plan a stop at the park's new visitor center, with its excellent informational display on the Occoneechee heritage and customs. William Townes established the 3,100-acre Occoneechee plantation on this site in 1839. As with many plantations, this was a virtually self-sustaining village until Townes's death in 1876, when the property was divided among his children and slaves. Eventually, the family sold the mansion, and it later burned to the ground in 1898.

After leaving US 58 to enter the park, you'll drive down VA 364, the park's main road. Turn left after the contact station and continue a short distance until you reach campground B on the right-hand side. There are 48 sites spread out over campgrounds B and C. The area once known as campground A was absorbed into the adjacent Occoneechee Wildlife Management Area. Sites are color-coded, so late arrivals should claim a vacant site of the same color and check in the following morning. Campground B is more RV oriented, and all 14 sites are open with hookups for RVs.

The entrance to campground C is farther down the park road on the right after you pass the 0.8-mile Big Oak Nature Trail. Many of the 35 sites located along dual loops

## :: Ratings

BEAUTY: ★ ★ ★ ★
SITE PRIVACY: ★ ★ ★ ★
SPACIOUSNESS: ★ ★ ★ ★
QUIET: ★ ★ ★
SECURITY: ★ ★ ★ ★
CLEANLINESS: ★ ★ ★ ★

# :: Key Information

**ADDRESS:** 1192 Occoneechee Park Road, Clarksville, VA 23927

**OPERATED BY:** Virginia Department of Conservation and Recreation

**CONTACT:** 434-374-2210; virginiastateparks.gov

**OPEN:** March 1–first Monday in December

**SITES:** 48

**SITE AMENITIES:** Picnic table, fire grill, lantern pole

**ASSIGNMENT:** On arrival as available

**REGISTRATION:** Call 800-933- PARK or visit reserveamerica.com; site assignment on arrival

**FACILITIES:** Equestrian campground, cabin rental, boat launch, fishing, playground, flush toilets, hot showers, laundry sinks

**PARKING:** At campsites, trailheads, and boat landing

**FEE:** $20–$23 per night; $27–$30 per night with electric/water hookups (prices vary depending on whether waterfront or inland); equestrian primitive campground $15 per night

**ELEVATION:** 350 feet

**RESTRICTIONS:**

■ **Pets:** Must be on a 6-foot or shorter leash; $5 per night

■ **Fires:** Only in camp stoves or fire rings

■ **Alcohol:** Public use or display is prohibited

■ **Vehicles:** Up to 35 feet; RV size limits are strictly enforced

■ **Other:** Maximum stay is 14 days in a 30-day period; maximum 6 people per site

on a small peninsula offer electric and water hookups and are located close together. Campground C is more tent oriented and would be the first choice for tent campers looking for quiet and privacy. It includes both primitive sites and sites with electric and water hookups. Tent pads are gravel, so plan to bring a sturdy ground cloth or tarp on which to pitch your tent. Plan to arrive during the week so that you can claim one of the sites with water views along the shoreline of campground C.

The equestrian campground is a fairly new addition to Occoneechee. It includes 11 100-foot-by-24-foot campsites with electricity and 11 12-foot-square covered stalls, which are not specifically assigned. Riding is allowed on the 7.5-mile Panhandle Multiuse Trail.

Besides the great fishing and boating that the John H. Kerr Reservoir has to offer, campers can enjoy a leisurely walk along the park's color-blazed trail system located between the contact station and entrance road to campground B. The trails range in length from the 1.2-mile Old Plantation Interpretive Trail to the 0.4-mile Warriors Path Nature Trail. Their degree of difficulty increases only as they dip and climb through riparian ravines. The park also offers picnic areas with excellent waterfront vistas. Swimming is not allowed from the park's shoreline.

Over the past couple of years, Virginia's state park system has been adding lodgings to those parks that did not have them. Be sure to check out this park's array of two- and three-bedroom cabins and two multibedroom lodges if you don't feel like roughing it.

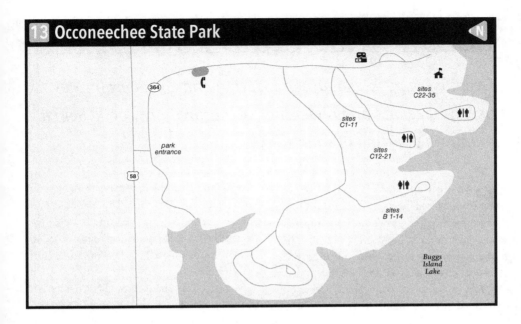

## :: Getting There

From I-85, take US 58 west at South Hill. Drive 20 miles until you spot the entrance for the park about 1 mile east of Clarksville.

**GPS COORDINATES**   N36° 38.146  W78° 31.758

# 14

# Pocahontas State Park

*Despite the park's suburban location and considerable day use, its size and preponderance of mature hardwoods help it maintain a feeling of sanctuary.*

**P**ocahontas State Park's 7,950 acres make it the largest park in the Virginia state park system, an especially impressive fact given that it lies a mere 20 miles from the state capital of Richmond. Indeed, the appeal of the park is not just its vast green space but also its convenient accessibility to residents of a major urban and suburban area. The park gets busy. During the summer you may find yourself bumping elbows with other campers and day users.

Whether you learned about Pocahontas through history class, legend, or the Disney animated movie, the name of this daughter of Chief Powhatan should be familiar to most. Legend has it that Pocahontas saved Captain John Smith from death at the hands of the Powhatan Confederacy, and later she married John Rolfe. The Powhatan version of the story is different. Regardless, there is little connection between the famous maiden and the park. It just happened to be the winning name suggested by a third-grader in a park-naming contest. The Civilian Conservation Corps built this, the first recreational park in the region, in the 1930s. The National Park Service operated what was originally known as the Swift Creek Recreation Area until 1946, when it was donated to the Commonwealth of Virginia.

Much has changed at this Chesterfield County location over the years, including a major campground reconstruction project. The original 34-site campground constructed by the CCC on a hillside along Swift Creek has given way to a larger facility with full electric and water hookups. While the quaintness of the former setting has been lost to us tent campers with the new, more RV-friendly campground, there are numerous sites that offer privacy and solitude. The preponderance of mature hardwoods helps maintain a feeling of sanctuary.

After turning off Beach Road at the park's entrance, you'll drive down the wide, forest-lined park road for a mile before reaching the contact station, after which you'll see the campground entrance on the right. The 114 campsites are situated along the main access road and loops A, B, and C against a dense backdrop of mature oaks with shorter holly and pine trees.

Hikers and mountain bikers can enjoy more than 80 miles of forest roads and trails that meander throughout the park. Some trails circle the 24-acre Beaver Lake, while others wind through the hardwood forest.

## :: Ratings

BEAUTY: ★ ★ ★ ★
SITE PRIVACY: ★ ★ ★
SPACIOUSNESS: ★ ★ ★
QUIET: ★ ★ ★
SECURITY: ★ ★ ★
CLEANLINESS: ★ ★ ★ ★

## :: Key Information

**ADDRESS:** 10301 State Park Road, Chesterfield, VA 23838-4713

**OPERATED BY:** Virginia Department of Conservation and Recreation

**CONTACT:** 804-796-4255; virginiastateparks.gov

**OPEN:** March–first Monday in December

**SITES:** 114

**SITE AMENITIES:** Picnic table, lantern pole, fire ring, electric/water hookups

**ASSIGNMENT:** First come, first served

**REGISTRATION:** Call 800-933-PARK or visit reserveamerica.com; site assignment on arrival

**FACILITIES:** Equestrian center, cabin rental, swimming pool, paddleboat launch, fishing, flush toilets, hot showers, pay phones, drink machines

**PARKING:** 1 vehicle and 1 camping unit per site; overflow near contact station

**FEE:** $27 per night; includes electric/water hookups

**ELEVATION:** 200 feet

**RESTRICTIONS:**
- **Pets:** $5 per night, on leash only
- **Fires:** In grills, camp stoves, or designated fire rings only
- **Alcohol:** Prohibited
- **Vehicles:** Up to 50 feet
- **Other:** Do not damage trees; no motorized vehicles on trails; swimming only in designated area; no gasoline motors on lake; maximum stay is 14 days in a 30-day period

Those out for a leisurely stroll will enjoy the 2.5-mile Beaver Lake Trail, and the 3.2-mile Old Mill Bicycle Trail offers an easy pedal through the park. Fat-tire bicyclists looking for a greater challenge will head for the three technical singletrack trails that were built as a joint effort between Pocahontas State Park and Mountain Bike Virginia bike club. Be sure to pick up copies of the *Pocahontas Park Guide* and *Bike Trails Guide*. There are also 9 miles of bridle paths for equestrian use on a BYOH (bring your own horse) basis.

Pocahontas State Park is also home to the Civilian Conservation Corps Museum. From 1933 to 1942, President Roosevelt responded to the Great Depression by creating an "army with shovels" that planted 2 billion trees and built roads, bridges, trails, and 800 state parks. The CCC Museum is housed in an original CCC building. Exhibits include letters, artifacts, photographs, and historic mementos that pay tribute to those whose contributions formed the most comprehensive conservation program ever known.

Whether you plan to hide out in the "wilds" of Chesterfield County or use Pocahontas State Park as a base camp from which to explore the city of Richmond, you're guaranteed to find this an inviting destination.

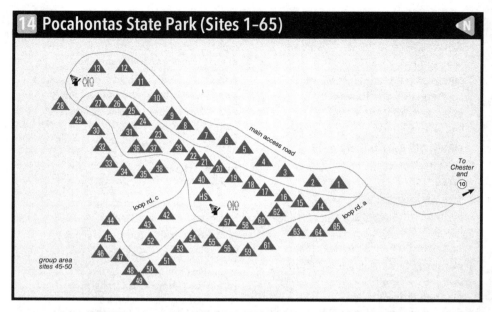

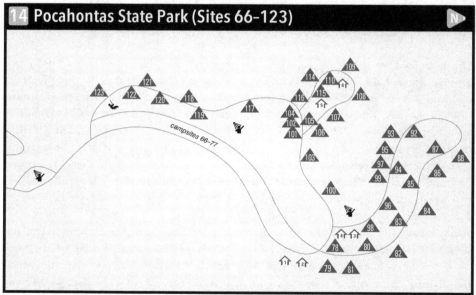

## :: Getting There

From I-95 take Exit 61 and go west on VA 10 past the village of Chester. Turn left onto Beach Road at the traffic light across from the old Chesterfield County Courthouse complex. Go 5 miles and turn right into the park's entrance.

**GPS COORDINATES**  N37° 22.476  W77° 34.631

# 15

# Smith Mountain Lake State Park

*The park is spread out over 1,248 densely wooded acres of Virginia pine, American beech, and juniper.*

**J**ust **35 miles** from Roanoke is the 20,000-acre, 50-mile-long Smith Mountain Lake. It's Virginia's second-largest freshwater lake. Bass anglers come from far and wide to land the citation largemouth and stripers that are caught every year during recreational and tournament fishing. A Virginia freshwater license is required whether fishing from the shore, a boat, or the fishing pier at the boat launch. Appalachian Power Company created the lake in 1960 by damming the Roanoke River, but the park didn't open until 1983. Smith Mountain Lake State Park is not just a fishing area, however. It is also a great destination for tent campers looking for a little solitude in the foothills of the Blue Ridge Mountains. In fact, if you remained at the campground during your entire stay, you'd never see the lake, which is rather inconspicuous unless you ride over to the Discovery Center, boat launch, or beachfront swimming area.

The 500-foot sandy beach is the park's only swimming area and features a

bathhouse and concessionaire, open during the summer. Paddleboats, Jet Skis, and pontoon boats are available for rent during this period. Other activities at Smith Mountain Lake State Park include guided night hikes, canoe trips, hayrides, bluegrass concerts, and twilight programs, in addition to popular junior ranger programs for children ages 6–10. Another popular spot is the picnic area located adjacent to the swimming area. Be sure to stop by the park's visitor center, where you'll find interesting exhibits describing area history, folklore, and environment.

The park is spread out over 1,248 densely wooded acres of Virginia pine, American beech, and juniper, which provide a back-to-nature feel while keeping the lake out of sight. The campground, visitor center, and boat launch and swimming area are situated on three separate peninsulas, so the best way to get from one to the other is by car. You can also reach the water by way of the trails, which range in length from the 0.5-mile Lake View Trail to the 1.9-mile Chestnut Ridge. Just outside the entrance to the visitor center is a kiosk and trailhead for the 1.3-mile Turtle Island Trail. The 0.5-mile Beechwood Trail is accessible from the dump station located next to the campground entrance. All of these trails provide easy to moderate excursions for hikers of average physical condition.

## :: Ratings

BEAUTY: ★ ★ ★
SITE PRIVACY: ★ ★
SPACIOUSNESS: ★ ★ ★
QUIET: ★ ★ ★
SECURITY: ★ ★ ★ ★
CLEANLINESS: ★ ★ ★

## :: Key Information

**ADDRESS:** 1235 State Park Road, Huddleston, VA 24104

**OPERATED BY:** Virginia Department of Conservation and Recreation

**CONTACT:** 540-297-6066; virginiastateparks.gov

**OPEN:** First weekend in March–Dec. 1

**SITES:** 50

**SITE AMENITIES:** Picnic table, fire ring, lantern post

**ASSIGNMENT:** First come, first served

**REGISTRATION:** Call 800-933-PARK or visit reserveamerica.com; site assignment on arrival

**FACILITIES:** Cabin and lodge rental; lake swimming, boating, and fishing; flush toilets; drink machine; hot showers; water; pay phone

**PARKING:** 1 vehicle per site, others at overflow parking area

**FEE:** Standard tent site $20 per night; $27 per night with electric/water hookups

**ELEVATION:** 920 feet

**RESTRICTIONS:**
- **Pets:** On short leash or enclosed; $3 per night
- **Fires:** In grills and fire rings only
- **Alcohol:** Public use or display is prohibited
- **Vehicles:** Up to 50 feet
- **Other:** Maximum stay is 14 days in a 30-day period; maximum 6 people, 2 tents per site; swimming in beach area only; quiet hours 10 p.m.–8 a.m.

After entering the park from VA 626, you'll see the modern visitor center on the right past the contact station. Turn left onto Interpretive Trail Road across from the office, and then turn left onto Overnight Road. You'll find the campground on the right, with overflow parking across the road. The campground consists of dual loops on which 50 sites are located. Sites 16–26, 27–35, and 42–47 lack hookups and are set off a short distance in the woods. Access to these sites requires a short walk from your car, but the additional privacy is worth it.

The other sites are located along the campground loop and set fairly close together. All sites are close to the new bathhouse, which is positioned in the center of the lower loop. Its flushing toilets and hot showers replaced the vault toilets in 2003. Like the rest of the park, the campground is set among a mixture of conifers and deciduous trees offering plentiful shade. Twenty en suite rental cabins are located nearby and feature docks and first-come, first-serve slips. With Smith Mountain Lake's popularity as a destination for bass anglers, it's especially advisable to plan your arrival during the week in the summer for optimum solitude.

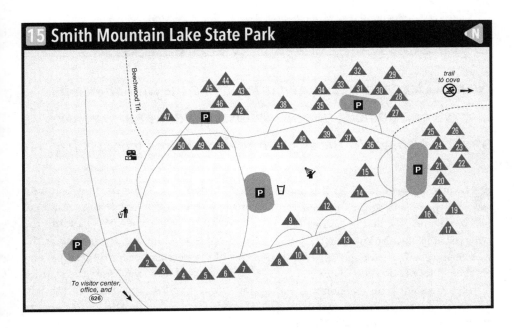

## :: Getting There

From Roanoke, head east on US 460 to Bedford. From there, proceed south on VA 122 to Moneta. Go east on VA 608, and then head south 2 miles on VA 626 to the park entrance.

**GPS COORDINATES**   N37° 04.972  W79° 35.611

# 16

# Staunton River State Park

*Nearby Occoneechee State Park may be the first choice for boaters and anglers, but the seclusion that Staunton River offers is well worth the 45-minute drive from Occoneechee.*

**S**taunton River State Park is located on a peninsula upstream from Occoneechee State Park at the narrow end of Buggs Island Lake, also known as the John H. Kerr Reservoir. The park and adjacent river are named for pre–Revolutionary War commander Captain Henry Staunton, whose contingent of soldiers kept early settlers safe from American Indian attacks. This section of the Dan River became known as Captain Dan's River and later the Staunton River. It became an important route for transporting tobacco from the large plantations that were built in this southernmost section of Virginia. Unfortunately, most were destroyed during the Civil War. This 1,597-acre park was one of the original six in Virginia's fledgling state park system. It opened in 1936, with many of the buildings constructed by the Civilian Conservation Corps from 1933 to 1935. Kerr Dam's opening in 1952 created the 48,000-acre Buggs Island Lake.

While nearby Occoneechee State Park may be the first choice for boaters

and anglers, the seclusion that Staunton River offers is well worth the 45-minute drive from Occoneechee. VA 344 forms the main park road before terminating at the end of the peninsula. Shortly after passing the contact station, you'll see the sign for Staunton River's campground on the left. Turn in here and enter the intimate figure eight where 48 sites are spread around a bathhouse in the center. Only 14 of these are standard sites without electric and water hookups, so, when things get busy, you're likely to have RVs for neighbors. The campground lies in a wooded enclave of oak and pine trees that provide a modicum of shade.

Chances are, however, that you'll spend little time in your tent when the sun is shining. Besides the aforementioned boating and fishing opportunities that attract many to Buggs Island Lake, bikers, hikers, and equestrians alike will enjoy the 7.5-mile River Bank Multi-Use Trail. The trail offers excellent water views and is an easy to moderate route that circumnavigates the 1,597-acre peninsula that's bounded by the Staunton and Dan rivers as well as Buggs Island Lake. It was developed as part of a concerted effort by the Virginia Department of Conservation and Recreation to accommodate a more diverse group of users, particularly mountain bikers. Other shorter trails range from 0.1 to 0.7 miles and serve to

## :: Ratings

BEAUTY: ★ ★ ★
SITE PRIVACY: ★ ★
SPACIOUSNESS: ★ ★
QUIET: ★ ★ ★
SECURITY: ★ ★ ★ ★
CLEANLINESS: ★ ★ ★ ★

## :: Key Information

**ADDRESS:** 1170 Staunton Trail, Scottsburg, VA 24589

**OPERATED BY:** Virginia Department of Conservation and Recreation

**CONTACT:** 434-572-4623; virginiastateparks.gov

**OPEN:** March–first Monday in December

**SITES:** 48

**SITE AMENITIES:** Picnic table, fire ring

**ASSIGNMENT:** On arrival

**REGISTRATION:** Call 800-933-PARK or visit reserveamerica.com; site assignment on arrival

**FACILITIES:** Equestrian campground, cabin rental, swimming pool, boat launch and fishing, laundry sinks, flush toilets, hot showers, drink machine, pay phone

**PARKING:** At campsites and day-use areas

**FEE:** Standard tent site $20 per night; $27 per night with electric/water hookups

**ELEVATION:** 370 feet

**RESTRICTIONS:**
■ **Pets:** On leash; $3 per night

■ **Fires:** In camp stove or fire ring only

■ **Alcohol:** Public use or display is prohibited

■ **Vehicles:** Up to 45 feet

■ **Other:** Quiet hours 10 p.m.–6 a.m.; maximum stay is 14 days in a 30-day period; maximum 6 people, 2 tents, and 2 vehicles per site

connect the park's main road with the River Bank Trail and other park facilities.

Horse folk will want to stop at the Equestrian Campground on the left before reaching the park contact station. It features 13 sites with electric and water hookups, 20 covered horse stalls, and a central dump station. Sites 1–10 are pull-through with paved surfacing and can accommodate a camping unit up to 50 feet long and one vehicle. Sites 11–13 are back-in with a gravel surface and can accommodate a camping unit up to 30 feet long with one vehicle. There is also a picnic shelter and a bathhouse with showers. Picnic tables, fire rings, and charcoal grills are available at each site.

Swimming from the park's shoreline is not allowed, but you'll be able to take a dip in the swimming pool after working up a sweat while playing tennis or mountain biking. The little ones will enjoy playground facilities located near the pool and tennis courts.

Enjoy a leisurely paddle on the surrounding waters in your canoe, or rent one from River Traders just west of the entrance to the park. Bird watchers will appreciate the bird checklist compiled over 20 years by Jeffrey Blalock. This list was updated in late 2003. It is available in the park office and lists the frequency of sightings by season.

For history buffs, Staunton River Battlefield State Park is a 20-minute drive away. Here, makeshift Confederate troops of old men and young boys held off 5,000 Union troops at a strategic railway bridge over the Staunton River. The 300-acre battlefield includes a modern visitor center that offers information about this historic site. Additionally, the roadbed of the former Richmond and Danville railroad line has reopened as a 0.8-mile walking trail from Staunton River bridge to Randolph.

Over the past couple of years, Virginia's state park system has been busy adding

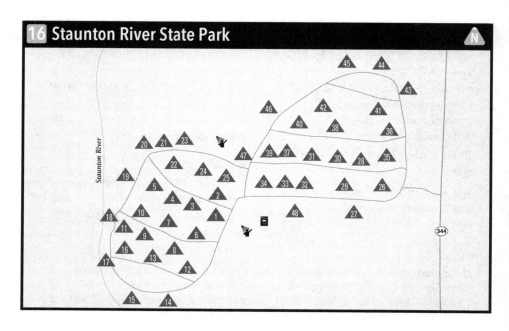

## 16 Staunton River State Park

lodgings to those parks that did not have them. While it may seem like blasphemy to inveterate tent campers, I have learned that age (and a bad back) is oft accompanied by an appreciation for indoor plumbing, a proper bed, and a hard roof, underneath which rain can actually be enjoyed. Be sure to check out this park's array of cabins and multibedroom lodges.

## :: Getting There

From US 58 along the southern border of Virginia, follow US 360 east 18 miles from South Boston. Turn right and continue 10 miles on VA 344 to the park entrance.

**GPS COORDINATES**   N36° 42.056 W78° 39.986

# 17

# Twin Lakes State Park

*The 6,970-acre Prince Edward–Gallion State Forest surrounds the park and offers an array of gated forest roads that are open to hikers and bikers.*

**L**ocated near Farmville in a shady area of mature hardwoods, Twin Lakes State Park is named for Goodwin Lake and Prince Edward Lake. The two lakes were in separate racially segregated parks that began operations in 1939 and continued in this fashion until the Civil Rights Act passed in 1964. The two integrated parks then operated separately until merging into one 425-acre park in 1976. The name was changed to Twin Lakes State Park in 1986. The park's main road and the 0.25-mile Between the Lakes Trail connect the two. Facilities at Goodwin Lake are available for individual camping, picnicking, and swimming. The eastern shore of Prince Edward Lake, meanwhile, features a lodge and cabins at the Cedar Crest Conference Center. The conference center is available by reservation only, with cabin rentals possible when not previously booked by groups.

After entering the park from VA 629, you'll find the campground located opposite the contact station. It consists of a large loop with a smaller loop at the rear. All of the sites are spacious, include water and electric hookups, and are set against a dense wooded background that provides ample shade during the summer. Sites 10 and 12, located at the back of the smaller loop that encompasses sites 6–15, are the most private of all. Tent pads are gravel, so pack a ground cloth for your tent and sleeping pad.

The day-use area at Goodwin Lake includes the 1-mile Goodwin Lake Nature Trail, a sandy beach, picnic tables, and a playground. The concession area, aka The Spot, is also located near here and offers bike rental, volleyball, horseshoes, camp items, and information. A relatively new addition to the park is the 14-mile Multi-Use Trail, which winds around through the adjacent 6,496-acre Prince Edward–Gallion State Forest. This trail is open to hikers, bikers, and equestrians.

Sometimes Twin Lakes' campground has sites available even when nearby Bear Creek Lake State Park and Holliday Lake State Park are full. Swimming is allowed on the designated beachfront area of Goodwin Lake, and the lakes can be used by boaters and anglers. A valid Virginia license is required for fishing. Canoes, kayaks, paddleboats, and rowboats are available for rent.

Pedestrian hiking trails range from the 0.25-mile, yellow-blazed Between the Lakes

## :: Ratings

BEAUTY: ★ ★ ★
SITE PRIVACY: ★ ★
SPACIOUSNESS: ★ ★ ★
QUIET: ★ ★ ★
SECURITY: ★ ★ ★
CLEANLINESS: ★ ★ ★

# :: Key Information

**ADDRESS:** 788 Twin Lakes Road, Green Bay, VA 23942

**OPERATED BY:** Virginia Department of Conservation and Recreation

**CONTACT:** 434-392-3435; virginiastateparks.gov

**OPEN:** March–first Monday in December

**SITES:** 33

**SITE AMENITIES:** Electricity, water, fire grill, picnic table

**ASSIGNMENT:** Your choice

**REGISTRATION:** Call 800-933-PARK or visit reserveamerica.com; site assignment on arrival

**FACILITIES:** Cabin rental; lake swimming, fishing, and boating; bathhouse; flush toilets; drink machine; pay phone

**PARKING:** 2 vehicles at campsite in addition to camping unit; additional parking at day-use area

**FEE:** $27 per night with electric/water hookups

**ELEVATION:** 450 feet

**RESTRICTIONS:**

■ **Pets:** $5 per night; keep on short leash or in enclosed area; no pets in lake

■ **Fires:** In grills, camp stoves, or designated fire rings only

■ **Alcohol:** Public use prohibited

■ **Vehicles:** Up to 36 feet

■ **Other:** Do not damage trees; maximum 6 people or 1 family per site; quiet hours 10 p.m.–6 a.m.; maximum stay is 14 days in a 30-day period

Trail to the fairly strenuous, orange-blazed, 4-mile Otter's Path Nature Trail that circles Prince Edward Lake. Also popular is the 1.5-mile, blue-blazed Goodwin Lake Nature Trail, which is less taxing and provides a number of interpretive signs describing the area's flora and fauna as it circles the smaller of the two lakes.

Prince Edward–Gallion State Forest surrounds the park and offers an array of gated forest roads that are open to hikers and bikers. Pick up a map of the forest, and plan an outing that will take you through an area that is home to raccoons, muskrats, white-tailed deer, wild turkey, and quail.

Cyclists, equestrians, and walkers may also want to leave Twin Lakes for a few hours to explore one of Virginia's newer parks, High Bridge Trail State Park. Located within a half-hour's drive and accessible from several spots near Farmville, this 31-mile linear rail bed last saw Norfolk Southern trains running in

2004, but the gentle 6% grade and crushed limestone surface is perfect for outdoor recreation.

Civil War buffs will want to visit nearby Sailor's Creek Battlefield Historical State Park, site of the last major battle of the Civil War. General Robert E. Lee's Army of Northern Virginia lost 7,700 men on April 6, 1865, leading to his surrender at Appomattox Court House 72 hours later. A former federal field hospital is open to the public in summer or by request; reenactments and encampments are but a portion of the "living history" at Sailor's Creek. A new visitor center houses exhibits whose timeline begins April 2, 1865, when Confederate forces left Richmond and Petersburg, and ends on April 8, 1865, the day prior to the surrender at Appomattox Court House. Displays also feature state-of-the-art holographic storytellers and artifacts from the battles at Sailor's Creek. It is part of Lee's

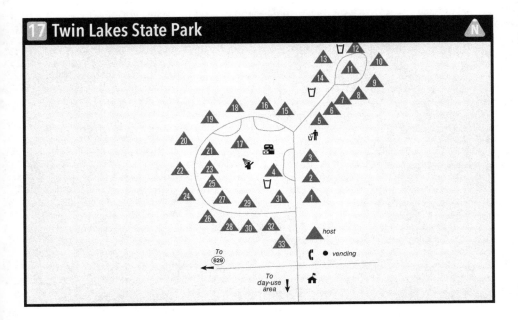

## 17 Twin Lakes State Park

Retreat Driving Tour, which goes from Petersburg to Appomattox, so you can tune to 1610 AM on your car radio to learn more about the events and battle that ended the Civil War.

## :: Getting There

From Richmond, drive west approximately 50 miles on US 360 through the town of Burkeville. Turn right onto VA 613 at the sign for Twin Lakes, and then turn right after a mile onto VA 629. Turn left into the campground entrance after driving 2 miles.

**GPS COORDINATES**  N37° 10.559  W78° 16.739

# Northern Virginia

# 18

# Bull Run Regional Park

*Civil War enthusiasts will readily identify Bull Run with the two battles fought at nearby Manassas National Battlefield Park.*

**B**ull **Run Regional Park** offers many things to those looking for some fresh air and respite from Northern Virginia gridlock. Civil War enthusiasts, however, will readily identify Bull Run with the two battles fought at nearby Manassas National Battlefield Park. Touring information can be found at the park's visitor center located on VA 234, which includes a bookstore offering an extensive array of Civil War titles. You can also pick up a battlefield map that details the various trails, roads, and sites that were part of First Manassas in July of 1861 and Second Manassas in August of 1862.

Follow the mile-long, self-guided walking tour of Henry Hill to see the First Manassas Battlefield. Located behind the visitor center, the tour uses recorded messages (accessed by cell phone) and signage to explain what occurred during this early clash between Confederate and Union troops on July 21, 1861. Union troops expected to take this strategic railroad junction and put an early end to the war. Such was the atmosphere of optimism that

citizens and congressmen from the capital arrived at the site literally prepared for a picnic. Confederate troops unexpectedly drove the Union soldiers back into Washington by 4 p.m., causing a chaotic situation as the retreating army got tangled up with sightseers. General Thomas J. Jackson received his nickname, "Stonewall," here, as he was reportedly observed to be standing in battle like a stone wall.

Thirty miles of hiking trails and 20 miles of bridle paths lace the 4,500-acre Manassas Battlefield. There is no connection between Bull Run Regional Park and the National Battlefield Park except proximity, but camping at Bull Run is a great way to gain access to this fascinating piece of U.S. and Virginia Civil War history.

Be sure to stop in the town of Manassas, especially at the visitor center located in the newly renovated train depot. A fascinating walking or driving tour of Old Town Manassas starts at the depot. In this designated Main Street Community, you'll find a wide selection of fine restaurants, art studios, galleries, and antiques shops, as well as the Manassas Volunteer Fire Company Museum. For day tours to Washington, D.C., leave your car in Manassas and catch a train. Request a parking permit from the visitor center, or leave from Manassas Park, where there are 677 spaces.

By the time you approach Bull Run Regional Park's entrance, the drone of I-66

## :: Ratings

BEAUTY: ★ ★ ★
SITE PRIVACY: ★ ★ ★ ★
SPACIOUSNESS: ★ ★ ★
QUIET: ★ ★ ★
SECURITY: ★ ★ ★ ★
CLEANLINESS: ★ ★ ★ ★

# :: Key Information

**ADDRESS:** 7700 Bull Run Drive, Centreville, VA 20121

**OPERATED BY:** Northern Virginia Regional Park Authority

**CONTACT:** 703-631-0550; nvrpa.org

**OPEN:** Year-round

**SITES:** 150

**SITE AMENITIES:** Picnic table, grill, campfire ring

**ASSIGNMENT:** First come, first served

**REGISTRATION:** Reservation on park website recommended, or on arrival

**FACILITIES:** Atlantis Waterpark, cabin rental, disc golf, equestrian trails, soccer fields, camp store, laundry, hot showers, playground, pay phone, water

**PARKING:** At campsites; max 2 vehicles per site

**FEE:** standard $26 per night; $30 per night with 30-amp electric hookup; $34.50 per night with 50-amp electric hookup; $39 per night with 30-amp service and full hookups; $43.50 with 50-amp service and full hookups; discounts for regional residents

**ELEVATION:** 160 feet

**RESTRICTIONS:**

■ **Pets:** Must be attended and on leash

■ **Fires:** Wood fires only within ground ring; only charcoal in grills; all fires must be attended; no collecting downed wood

■ **Alcohol:** Prohibited

■ **Vehicles:** Up to 45 feet

■ **Other:** Quiet hours 10 p.m.–7 a.m.; maximum stay of 7 consecutive days; maximum of 7 campers per site, with additional fee charged after 4 campers per site

will have wafted off into the background. Drive 2 more miles to reach the campground and you'll get an idea of the park's other offerings, including picnic shelters; minigolf and disc golf courses; soccer fields; a large swimming pool; a wildlife-viewing bench by a water hole; and a shooting center featuring skeet, archery, and a sporting clay course. The expansive, grassy playing fields and sycamore trees on the park's 1,500 flat acres bordering Cub Run and Bull Run suggest a floodplain, but the campground is located on higher ground with its own emergency access, so high water is generally not a problem.

The heavily wooded campground is located near the center of the park. Sites are well spaced, private, flat, and spread out along a large loop with three smaller inner loops. A third of the 150 sites are nonelectric; these are located along the outer edge of the campground loop. While campers may have particular preferences on arrival, the combination of dense oak woods, understory, and ample size and spacing of campsites is such that you'll have a hard time finding fault with any of the nonelectric sites. Municipal parks must be many things to many people, but Bull Run's ability to provide such a pleasant back-to-the-woods camping experience within a stone's throw of I-66 and Washington, D.C., is nothing short of amazing. The park readily fills up on holiday weekends as well as in early spring, when Bull Run's famous bluebells are in bloom. Reservations are recommended at all times.

Nature trails traverse the area, but hikers and equestrians looking for an extended outing will head for the 17.5-mile (point-to-point) Bull Run Occoquan Trail; the trailhead is located near the campground entrance. Winding along the Occoquan Reservoir through 4,000 acres of riparian

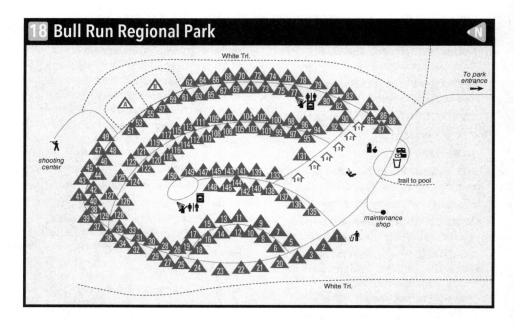

woodlands, this linear trail passes Hemlock Overlook Park and Bull Run Marina before reaching its terminus at Fountainhead Park.

Be sure to pick up a trail brochure for more information before starting out.

## :: Getting There

From I-66, take Exit 52 at Centreville, and go 2 miles south on US 29 to Bull Run Post Office Road. Follow signs to the park entrance at a sharp bend to the left.

**GPS COORDINATES**   N38° 48.278  W77° 28.711

# 19

# Burke Lake Park

*You don't need to jump back into your vehicle to find something to do after setting up your campsite.*

**E**ntering **Burke Lake Park** from Ox Road in Fairfax County, the first impression you'll have is of the park's 18-hole golf course and driving range. Keep driving, however, as the park's main road winds around past the 218-acre lake before reaching the campground entrance located next to the maintenance area. Burke Lake Road is an alternate, albeit less picturesque, entrance to the campground.

The campground's 120 sites, none with electric hookups, are spread out among areas A, B, and C. There is a noticeable difference among sites, so campers should drive or walk through the campground before choosing a site. For those of us who crave a little privacy in the woods, sites B1–16 are the most appealing, with 4, 6, 8, and 10 at the top of the list because they are the most private and border the park's 5-mile trail.

Someone has long since given up on the idea of growing any vegetation under the trees in C, so all that remains is a gravel base. As a result, those sites in area C were hard to distinguish from each other or, for that matter,

from the gravel roads that loop throughout this section of the 883-acre park. There are some appealing sites in area A, but these are in close proximity to the group-camping area and the entrance road to the campground, allowing for the possibility of somewhat noisy conditions. Groups of seven or more campers can use the wilderness camping area, which will get you as far into the woods as possible at Burke Lake Park. Note that the wilderness camping area, however, is primitive and lacks water and restroom facilities. The wilderness area includes an orienteering course laid out for both beginners and advanced map and compass users.

The beauty of camping at Northern Virginia campgrounds like Burke Lake is not so much the ability to rough it but more the opportunity to sleep outdoors while taking advantage of all the recreational, cultural, and educational activities that this vast suburb of Washington, D.C., has to offer. Don't think, however, that you need to jump back into your vehicle to find something to do after setting up your campsite. Therein lies the key to enjoying this facility managed by the Fairfax County Park Authority.

The 218-acre lake itself offers myriad possibilities. Whether you bring your own canoe or rent a boat on site, you're sure to enjoy exploring Burke Lake's interesting coves, as well as the waterfowl refuge on Vesper Island, which lies within its boundaries. Gasoline motors and sailboats are not allowed

## :: Ratings

BEAUTY: ★ ★ ★
SITE PRIVACY: ★ ★ ★
SPACIOUSNESS: ★ ★ ★
QUIET: ★ ★
SECURITY: ★ ★ ★
CLEANLINESS: ★ ★ ★

## :: Key Information

| | |
|---|---|
| **ADDRESS:** 7315 Ox Road, Fairfax Station, VA 22039 | **PARKING:** Limited to 1 camping vehicle and 1 other vehicle |
| **OPERATED BY:** Fairfax County Park Authority | **FEE:** $28 per night; discounts for seniors 65 and older |
| **CONTACT:** 703-323-6600; fairfaxcounty.gov/parks/burkelakepark | **ELEVATION:** 430 feet |
| **OPEN:** Mid-April–October | **RESTRICTIONS:** |
| **SITES:** 120 | ■ **Pets:** Must be on leash |
| **SITE AMENITIES:** Picnic table and grill | ■ **Fires:** Wood fires in ring only; charcoal fire in grill; wood gathering prohibited |
| **ASSIGNMENT:** First come, first served | ■ **Alcohol:** Prohibited |
| **REGISTRATION:** On site | ■ **Vehicles:** Up to 25 feet |
| **FACILITIES:** Miniature and 18-hole golf courses, lake boating, playgrounds, fishing, ice cream parlor, camp store, hot showers, water, pay phone | ■ **Other:** Maximum stay is 14 days; quiet time 10 p.m.–7 a.m.; all campers must use a camper, tent, or other camping device; cannot bring firewood from outside the D.C. area |

on the lake. Many Northern Virginian anglers come to the lake to cast a line for largemouth bass, walleye, muskie, catfish, crappie, perch, and bluegill. Bait and tackle are available at the park's marina, or bring your own. Virginia fishing licenses are required.

Picnic areas with shelters for rent, an 18-hole par-three golf course, a driving range, a disc golf course, a miniature railroad, a 5-mile walking trail, an 18-station fitness trail, sand volleyball courts, playing fields, and even an ice-cream parlor are the kinds of activities that you'll find at this island of green amid the sprawling developments of Northern Virginia. There is no pool, and swimming is not allowed in the lake. Don't let this discourage you, however,

as campers wanting pools will head to Lake Fairfax or Pohick, leaving Burke Lake to you. It's enough to keep you having outdoor fun for days, but if you are camping at Burke Lake with the intent of touring the surrounding area, hop in the car for a short drive over to Mount Vernon, Woodlawn Plantation, and George Washington's Grist Mill. The nation's capital is around 20 miles away, but Northern Virginia's rush hour traffic is legendary and parking is scarce in D.C. Fight the urge to drive in—park your car at the Springfield Metrorail lot or Burke Center Virginia Rail Express lot, and take the train. The Burke Lake Camp Store hands out photocopied driving directions to the Metro, so be sure to ask.

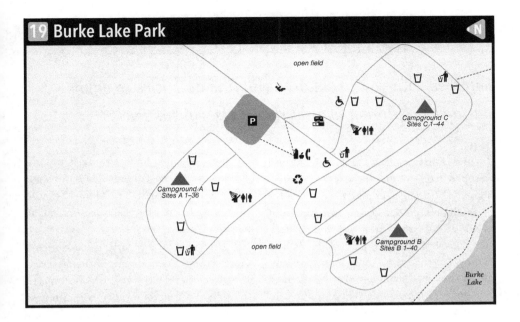

## :: Getting There

From the I-495 Beltway, take Exit 5 onto Braddock Road. Go west on Braddock Road, and then turn left onto Ox Road. Drive a short distance until you see the park entrance on the left.

**GPS COORDINATES** N38° 46.135 W77° 18.089

# 20

# Lake Fairfax Park

*Families with young children will find activities to enjoy during the summer at suburban Lake Fairfax Park.*

**L**ake Fairfax Park's 476 wooded and open acres are tucked away in a unique, high-end planned community in the suburbs of Washington, D.C. Reston was conceived as a spacious urban area with a rural feel, complete with protected parks and greenery. Planners in the 1960s could never have predicted the high-tech boom that has flooded Northern Virginia with dense traffic and urban sprawl; nevertheless, their foresight has preserved the forested environment that made Reston so desirable. Lake Fairfax is located near I-495, I-66, and VA 7, but you'd never know it as you drive down the wooded approach off Baron Cameron Avenue.

The first thing you'll notice as you enter the park is the Water Mine Family Swimming Hole. Campers receive reduced rates at the attraction, which includes waterslides, flumes, sprinklers, and floatables. You may scoff at this commercialism that obviously does not make for the ideal wilderness experience, but families with kids who are just breaking into camping will find that the Water Mine makes the experience a

lot more palatable for the youngsters. And in the summer, most of us will find the water attraction downright refreshing because swimming has not been allowed in the lake for several years.

Driving into the park, you'll notice a more natural environment with tree-lined streams alongside the road, which climbs to the hilltop campground. You will also pass signs for the requisite ball fields, as in any other Northern Virginia municipal park. In addition, Lake Fairfax Park offers a cricket field—a testament to Northern Virginia's multicultural population. The camp store features a recent-sightings board where you may find that, in addition to softball players and swimmers, foxes, turkey buzzards, skunks, deer, turkeys, woodchucks, and owls have been spotted nearby.

Most of the campsites have electric hookups, and many are in the open field with a few oak trees scattered about. Along the wooded edge, however, are a number of sites that provide shade and privacy. Plan your arrival during the week, and take a close look at those attractive sites hugging the western edge of camping area A.

As with other Northern Virginia municipal campgrounds, camping at Fairfax Lake Park is not the ultimate back-to-nature experience that many would imagine, but it's ideal for the family who is trying out tent camping while keeping a wide array of less woodsy entertainment close by. Other

## :: Ratings

BEAUTY: ★ ★ ★
SITE PRIVACY: ★ ★ ★
SPACIOUSNESS: ★ ★ ★
QUIET: ★ ★ ★
SECURITY: ★ ★ ★
CLEANLINESS: ★ ★ ★

## :: Key Information

**ADDRESS:** 1400 Lake Fairfax Drive, Reston, VA 20190

**OPERATED BY:** Fairfax County Park Authority

**CONTACT:** 703-471-5415; fairfaxcounty.gov/parks/lakefairfax

**OPEN:** Year-round

**SITES:** 72 individual sites and 9 group camping areas

**SITE AMENITIES:** Picnic table, grill/fire ring

**ASSIGNMENT:** First come, first served

**REGISTRATION:** By reservation at 703-471-5415; call 703-757-9242 May–September

**FACILITIES:** Water Mine water park, skate park, lake boating and fishing, playground, hot showers, flush toilets, camp store

**PARKING:** 1 vehicle in addition to camping unit

**FEE:** $28 per night; $37 per night for tent or pop-up with 20/30-amp service; $45 per night for RV/trailer with 20/30/50-amp service (up to 4 people), $2 per night additional person to maximum of 7; discounts available for Fairfax residents and seniors 65 and older

**ELEVATION:** 520 feet

**RESTRICTIONS:**

■ **Pets:** On leash and attended at all times

■ **Fires:** In camp stove, grill, or fireplace only; no wood in charcoal grills; only wood from D.C. area can be brought in

■ **Alcohol:** Prohibited

■ **Vehicles:** No limit

■ **Other:** Maximum stay during summer is 14 days, 28 days Labor Day–Memorial Day; quiet time 10 p.m.–7 a.m.; campers must use a camper, tent, or other camping device.

books have been written about all that there is to do in this vast suburb of Washington, D.C., and no doubt many will find that Lake Fairfax Park is an ideal and relatively inexpensive place to stay while sightseeing around our nation's capital. Just leave your car at Vienna or West Falls Church station and take the Metrorail into the District. You could, however, just as easily leave your cell phone and laptop at home, park your car, and enjoy the park's activities without driving again until you've broken camp.

Lake Fairfax Park also features a playground, a carousel, short trails, and a miniature train ride. In addition, you can fish and rent paddleboats to laze around the 18-acre lake. You can drop your line for panfish in the lake or stocked trout in the stream that courses through the park. There is even a free children's entertainment series held on Saturdays throughout the summer. Undoubtedly, Lake Fairfax Park offers a different sort of camping and outdoor experience than most others in this guide. But this is Northern Virginia, and families with children will find a lot to enjoy during the summer at Lake Fairfax Park.

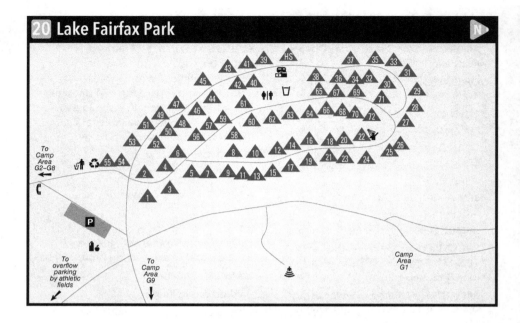

## :: Getting There

From the I-495 Beltway, take Exit 47A west 6.5 miles. Turn left onto Baron Cameron Avenue (VA 606) and then left onto Lake Fairfax Drive. The park entrance is a short distance ahead.

**GPS COORDINATES**   N38° 57.739  W77° 19.268

# 21

# Pohick Bay Regional Park

*Even landlubbers will find these 150 campsites great places to sleep under the trees.*

**P**ohick was named by Algonquin Indians to aptly describe this area as the "water place." With its marina, boat launch, and boat storage facilities, Pohick Bay Regional Park offers a year-round haven for boaters looking for access to the Potomac River, just 25 miles south of Washington, D.C., in Fairfax County. Those without a boat can choose from the park's rental fleet of paddleboats, sailboats, and johnboats. Even landlubbers will find Pohick Bay's 150 campsites great places to sleep under the trees while leaving Northern Virginia's traffic jams behind.

After entering the park from Gunston Road, turn right and follow the signs to reach the camping area. Once you reach the camp center and store, continue straight to reach sites 1–100 (with hookups), or go left for 101–150 (sans electricity). Both spots offer flat sites in a nicely wooded area laden with pine, beech, and holly trees. Do not automatically skip those sites with hookups because you don't need electricity. You might find them desirable if the park is busy. If you decide to go this route, try to get one of sites 31–38, which form a small loop at the back of a much larger loop composed of the remaining sites with electricity; these encircle a grassy playing field and offer a considerable degree of privacy. The sites without electric hookups are located a short distance away on the opposite side of the park's disc golf course and popular, large swimming pool. These are also laid out on a bigger and smaller loop in a more contained but heavily wooded area. Sites 101–150 appear smaller than 1–100 with more understory between sites, so the privacy issue is probably a wash. Should you camp in the nonelectric area, try to get one of sites 103–120, which are spacious and offer a good deal of privacy. Weekends and holidays are busy times at Pohick, especially given its emphasis on boating activities, so try to plan a midweek outing if solitude and silence are high on your priority list.

Municipal parks such as this one take a different approach to outdoor recreation than the state and federal campgrounds listed in this guide. There are probably those purists who would eschew camping in a facility that features 18-hole golf and disc golf courses, expansive playing fields, and boating facilities—everybody is entitled to his own definition of back to nature. But this model, which includes the Pirate's Cove Waterpark, is better able to meet the recreational needs of more than 3 million

## :: Ratings

BEAUTY: ★ ★ ★
SITE PRIVACY: ★ ★ ★
SPACIOUSNESS: ★ ★ ★
QUIET: ★ ★ ★
SECURITY: ★ ★ ★
CLEANLINESS: ★ ★ ★

## :: Key Information

| | |
|---|---|
| **ADDRESS:** 6501 Pohick Bay Drive, Lorton, VA 22709 | **PARKING:** At campsite and swimming pool |
| **OPERATED BY:** Northern Virginia Regional Park Authority | **FEE:** $26 per night; electric site $28 per night (up to 4 campers), $3 per additional person; full-hookup site $43.50; discounts for regional residents |
| **CONTACT:** 703-339-6104; nvrpa.org | |
| **OPEN:** Year-round | |
| **SITES:** 150 | **ELEVATION:** 50 feet |
| **SITE AMENITIES:** Picnic table and grill; 100 have electric hookup | **RESTRICTIONS:** |
| **ASSIGNMENT:** First come, first served | ▓ **Pets:** Must be attended and on leash shorter than 6 feet |
| **REGISTRATION:** Reservation on park website and on arrival | ▓ **Fires:** In camp stove and fire ring only; no collecting deadwood |
| **FACILITIES:** Lake paddling, Pirate's Cove Waterpark, golf course, disc golf, minigolf, playground, camp store, laundry, soda machine, pay phone, water, showers | ▓ **Alcohol:** Prohibited |
| | ▓ **Vehicles:** Site specific up to 50 feet |
| | ▓ **Other:** Maximum 7 campers per site; 14-day maximum stay; quiet hours 10 p.m.–7 a.m. |

Northern Virginians than a more remote campground would be, and it keeps families from having to spend the better part of a weekend driving to find a campsite.

Pohick Bay is close to Mount Vernon, Gunston Hall, and other regional attractions. Those wishing to take a day trip into Washington, D.C., should either drive 5.3 miles to the Lorton Virginia Rail Express station or 11 miles to the Springfield Metro. Inquire at the camp store about guided bus tours.

If you're looking for more nature-oriented activities to enjoy during your stay at Pohick, take a short drive down Gunston Road to Mason Neck State Park. This wildlife refuge has more than 200 species of birds. You'll see more than 1,000 pairs of great blue herons in their rookery, a scene that appears almost prehistoric as these massive birds croak at each other and gently flap through the air with their necks bent. But it's the 15–50 bald eagles that frequent the park that attract many birding enthusiasts.

## :: Getting There

From I-95, take the Exit 163 (Lorton). Turn left onto Lorton Road, right onto US 1, and then left onto Gunston Road. Continue past the golf course to the park entrance on the left.

**GPS COORDINATES**   N38° 40.239  W77° 10.497

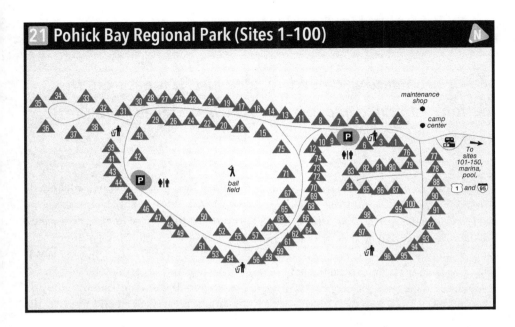

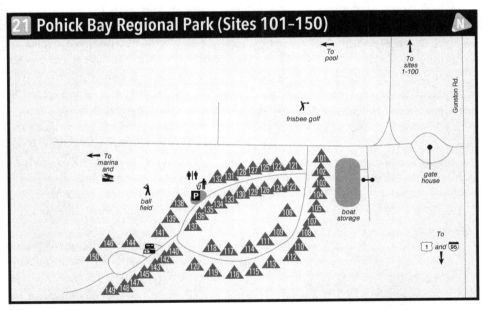

# 22

# Prince William Forest Park

*This 17,000-acre woodland, located just 32 miles from the nation's capital, could just as easily be 32 miles from the middle of nowhere.*

**I**f **your** perception of Northern Virginia is traffic gridlock, rampant development, and trees as endangered species, then Prince William Forest Park may very well cause an abrupt mind-shift. This 17,000-acre woodland, located just 32 miles from the nation's capital, could just as easily be 32 miles from the middle of nowhere. Once you've gotten to the Oak Ridge Campground in the northwestern corner of the park, the bustle and sounds of I-95 shadowing the park's entrance on the eastern edge will have long since drifted away.

The park's history dates back thousands of years to those days when Algonquin-speaking American Indians hunted and fished here prior to the arrival of the first European settlers in 1607. This Chesapeake Bay watershed saw expansive tobacco cultivation and pyrite mining before benefiting from Civilian Conservation Corps labor and gaining national forest status in 1936. Although developed for recreational usage

and watershed protection, the park became home to the Office of Strategic Services, the precursor to the Central Intelligence Agency, during World War II. In 1945, Prince William reverted to public use following WWII and remains the largest natural area in the Washington, D.C., metropolitan region and the largest area of piedmont forest in the national park system.

After leaving I-95 at Exit 150, follow the signs a short distance to the park's entrance. Stop by the visitor center, pick up a map of the park, and take in the exhibit explaining the rich history of Prince William Forest Park before heading off to the Oak Ridge Campground. The campground is 5.5 miles from the visitor center along the paved scenic drive. Plan to have the $20 per night camping fee in exact change ready so that, once you've pitched your tent, you're good to go. Once you've made it to this oasis, you'll not want to use your car again until it's time to go.

The Oak Ridge Campground consists of three loops, A, B, and C, with nary a hookup among the 100 sites. RVs will have motored to the Prince William RV Campground on the other side of the park, so you're not likely to run up against somebody's Minnie Winnie. Campers may collect dead and downed firewood less than 6 inches in diameter.

The overall terrain is rolling, but the campground itself is private, flat, and heavily

## :: Ratings

BEAUTY: ★ ★ ★ ★
SITE PRIVACY: ★ ★ ★ ★
SPACIOUSNESS: ★ ★ ★ ★
QUIET: ★ ★ ★ ★
SECURITY: ★ ★ ★ ★
CLEANLINESS: ★ ★ ★

## :: Key Information

**ADDRESS:** 18100 Park Headquarters Road, Triangle, VA 22172

**OPERATED BY:** National Park Service

**CONTACT:** 703-221-7181; nps.gov/prwi

**OPEN:** Year-round

**SITES:** 100

**SITE AMENITIES:** Picnic table, grill, lantern pole

**ASSIGNMENT:** First come, first served on loop A (April–October)

**REGISTRATION:** Self-registration on site; reservations for loops B and C at recreation.gov

**FACILITIES:** Cabin rental, water, flush toilets, shower in loop B, hot showers at Oak Ridge, bike rack

**PARKING:** 2 vehicles per site, additional vehicles park at campground entrance

**FEE:** $20 per night; free at Chopawamsic Backcountry area

**ELEVATION:** 350 feet

**RESTRICTIONS:**
▇ **Pets:** On 6-foot leash

▇ **Fires:** In grills; bring your own USDA-certified pest-free firewood; collect downed deadwood within campground area for use during stay

▇ **Alcohol:** At campsite

▇ **Vehicles:** Up to 32 feet for campers and up to 26 feet for trailers

▇ **Other:** Quiet hours 10 p.m.– 6 a.m.; maximum 6 people and 2 tents per site; 14-day maximum stay; fireworks, firearms, and weapons prohibited

wooded with second-growth oaks and some small pines. Sites vary in size from spacious in loops A and B to the extremely spacious walk-in sites in loop C. The campground rarely fills up. Some use it as a relatively inexpensive way to explore Washington, but my feeling is that it's too beautiful and natural a setting to park and drive away. There are several Northern Virginia campgrounds that are closer to D.C., but if you opt to use Prince William as your base camp for urban exploration, avoid rush hour on I-95 by taking the Virginia Rail Express from nearby Rippon or Quantico to D.C.'s Union Station.

Opportunities for bikers and hikers abound at this park. Some 37 miles of well-blazed hiking trails with varied lengths and degrees of difficulty wind through the beech, holly, and oak forest. The best place to start might be the 1-mile Farms to Forest Trail (with a possible 2.7-mile extension through

beaver habitat), which begins right at the campground entrance. From the 0.2-mile Pine Grove Forest Trail to the 9.7-mile South Valley Trail, there's something for anyone who wants to take a walk in the woods.

The park is also bicycle-friendly, whether you're on a road bike or mountain bike. The 7.5-mile paved scenic loop includes a 3-mile section of separate bike lanes from parking lot D to the Oak Ridge Campground. There are also 9.2 miles of fire roads for mountain bikers that are rated from easy to difficult. The trails, however, are closed to bicycles, so many of these fire roads are out-and-back rides. Be sure to pick up a copy of the bicycling guide from the visitor center.

Whether you're looking for a respite from the hectic pace of Northern Virginia or a wooded destination at which to spend a few days, you'll find your time at Prince William Forest Park to be absolutely rejuvenating.

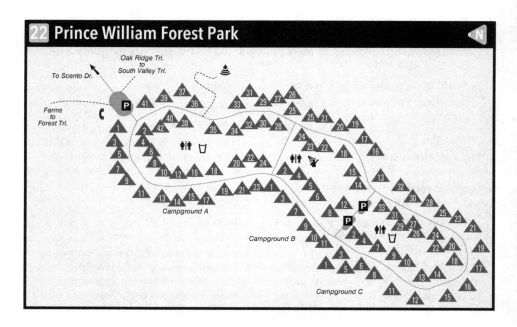

## :: Getting There

From I-95, take Exit 150 or 150B to VA 619 West. Follow the signs less than 1 mile to the park's entrance.

**GPS COORDINATES** N38° 35.946 W77° 25.038

# Western Virginia

# 23

# Big Meadows Campground

*You're likely to see white-tailed deer, song sparrows, meadowlarks, grouse, foxes, and skunks.*

**B**ig **Meadows** is Shenandoah National Park's largest treeless area, encompassing a barren plateau that is approximately 640 acres. It's believed that American Indians cleared the area to create favorable grazing conditions. European settlers overgrazed this site with beef cattle, especially during the Civil War. Park officials have waged an ongoing battle against the growth of black locust and blackberry that would, if left unchecked, take over the meadow. In the past, Park Service officials used combinations of burning and mowing to hold back the growth of invasive vegetation. New strategies have aided in the establishment of meadow grasses. Today, the dominant shrub growth in the meadow is blueberry, with swamp varieties, such as marsh marigold, swamp fern, and Canadian burnet, growing in wetter areas. Overall, the meadow supports some 270 species of vascular plants. In addition to the white-tailed deer that wander seemingly carefree through the meadow, you're also likely to see song sparrows, meadowlarks, grouse, foxes, and skunks.

## :: Ratings

BEAUTY: ★ ★ ★ ★

SITE PRIVACY: ★ ★ ★ ★

SPACIOUSNESS: ★ ★ ★ ★

QUIET: ★ ★ ★ ★

SECURITY: ★ ★ ★ ★

CLEANLINESS: ★ ★ ★ ★ ★

The park's dedication was held at Big Meadows, the spiritual center of Skyline Drive, on July 3, 1936. President Franklin D. Roosevelt himself was on hand to formally open the facilities at Shenandoah National Park. The meadow is located across Skyline Drive from the Harry F. Byrd Visitor Center, which houses informative exhibits, a library, an auditorium, interpretive programs, and an array of literature about Shenandoah National Park that is on sale in the small gift shop. Be sure to pick up a copy of *Explore Shenandoah*, the park's newsletter, for a great overview of where things are located in Shenandoah National Park as well as times and locations for ranger programs.

Big Meadows, with its visitor center, lodge, restaurant, and campground, is located in the central section of the park at mile 51.2. After pulling off Skyline Drive near the Byrd Visitor Center, follow the signs to the registration station for Big Meadows Campground. Its 217 sites are situated on two large loops, the front one containing loops P–T, and the rear section containing U–Y. Except for sites 1–53, which are tents only, all are designated RV sites, despite the lack of hookups.

The sites are spacious and separated by considerable foliage. Park officials did a good job of placing a large number of sites close to each other without sacrificing seclusion. This is, of course, relative; those of you who relish your solitude will accept the

## :: Key Information

**ADDRESS:** Skyline Drive, milepost 51

**OPERATED BY:** National Park Service

**CONTACT:** 540-999-3500, ext. 3231; nps.gov

**OPEN:** Weather dependent; spring–late autumn

**SITES:** 217

**SITE AMENITIES:** Picnic table, fire grill

**ASSIGNMENT:** On arrival by camper; assigned on busy weekends

**REGISTRATION:** By reservation at recreation.gov or on arrival

**FACILITIES:** Camp store, laundry, coin-operated showers, lodge with restaurant

**PARKING:** At campsites and at laundry and shower area

**FEE:** $20 per night, plus $15 park entrance; discounts for holders of Interagency Senior/Access passes and Golden Age/Access passes

**ELEVATION:** 3,600 feet

**RESTRICTIONS:**

■ **Pets:** On 6-foot leash or shorter; clean up after pet

■ **Fires:** Only in camp stoves and fireplaces

■ **Alcohol:** Permitted

■ **Vehicles:** No limit

■ **Other:** Do not damage any trees; wash dishes at campsite only; discard gray water in service sinks at restrooms; maximum 6 people, 2 tents, 2 vehicles per site; quiet hours 10 p.m.–6 a.m.; noise limit for generators and use restricted to 8–10 a.m. and 4–7 p.m.

slight inconvenience of walking 10–100 yards and opt for one of the walk-to sites.

The walk-to sites are set off in the wooded edge of Big Meadows Campground and are very private. Sites 1–8 are set between the main entrance road and the camp road and tend to be noisier than the others, but appealing sites 29–34 and 44–53 are set off by themselves in the woods. Sites 12–21 and 24–34 are in grassy and less wooded areas but are still highly desirable if you don't mind carrying your gear a short distance to your site. There are no sites 25 and 26. Big Meadows Campground is a popular stopover for campers in Shenandoah National Park, especially in the fall, and it is the only one that accepts reservations. If you can plan your stay during the week, you'll find considerably fewer neighbors, but calling ahead is a good idea at any time.

As in the rest of this nearly 300-square-mile park through which 101 miles of the famed Appalachian Trail passes, there is no shortage of hiking trails. However, the Big Meadows area is especially blessed with trails for hikers of varied ages and ability levels. The 1.8-mile Story of the Forest Nature Trail is a relatively easy walk starting from the Byrd Visitor Center. Interpretive signs explain various aspects of the surrounding forest. The 3.3-mile Lewis Falls Trail provides more of a challenge in terms of length and change in elevation after it exits the amphitheater parking lot. The hike to the 81-foot falls is worth the effort.

Camp Hoover (aka Rapidan Camp), located across from Big Meadows 6.3 miles down the Rapidan Fire Road, was a favorite getaway for President Herbert Hoover. The walk to Camp Hoover can be shortened to a 4-mile out-and-back by taking the Mill Prong Trail. Camp Hoover is a beautiful spot where 3 of the original 13 cabins remain at the confluence of Mill Prong, Laurel Prong,

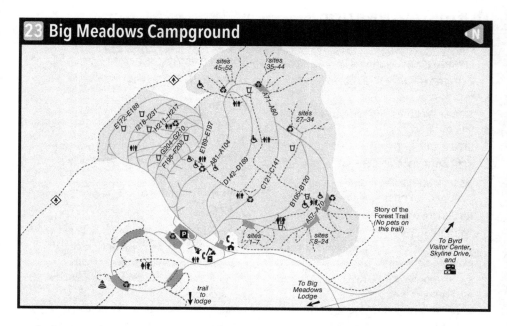

## 23 Big Meadows Campground

and the Rapidan River. In the summer, three-hour van tours are available several days a week. Sign up in advance at the Byrd Visitor Center. While many campers make their pilgrimage to Shenandoah National Park in the fall when colors are at their most varied and brightest, May represents the peak time for wildflowers in the meadow.

## :: Getting There

From the Swift Run Gap Entrance Station at mile 65.7, drive north on Skyline Drive to Big Meadows at mile 51.2.

**GPS COORDINATES**  N38° 31.709 W78° 26.334

# 24

# Camp Roosevelt Recreation Area

*You'd be hard-pressed to find quieter and larger campsites anywhere.*

**T**he single greatest conservation movement in history began on March 31, 1933, when President Franklin D. Roosevelt created the Civilian Conservation Corps in response to the Great Depression. The goal was twofold: to put the nation's young men back to work and to conserve forests and natural environments.

A month later, the first enrollees of "Roosevelt's boys" marched into the George Washington National Forest and broke ground on the inaugural CCC camp—Camp Roosevelt. FDR's "army with shovels" went on to plant 2 billion trees and build roads, bridges, trails, and 800 state parks. The results of their work can be admired throughout the country, but locally CCC work endures along Skyline Drive, Fort Valley, and throughout national parks and forests. By the time World War II arrived, 3 million men were ardent conservationists.

It is fitting, then, that the campground at Camp Roosevelt is peaceful, undeveloped, and wooded. The 10 campsites are spacious

with plenty of vegetation and land between them. You'd be hard-pressed to find quieter and larger campsites anywhere.

Camp Roosevelt is located a short distance from Massanutten Mountain at the lower end of Fort Valley and a short distance from the Lee Ranger District Office in Edinburg. The entrance to the recreation area is at the intersection of FDR 274 and VA 675, with the picnic area straight ahead and the campground to the left. The campground loop is arranged around a grassy central area where the bathhouse is located, and the entire site is co-located with the old CCC barracks and recreation hall. Adjacent to the campground is a picnic area where you'll find foundations from some early CCC buildings. There is also a memorial to Henry Rich, the first man inducted into the CCC, and a plaque commemorating historic Camp Roosevelt as the first CCC camp. Camp Roosevelt CCC alumni returned to the site and constructed the group picnic shelter in 1983.

One way to explore and get to know more about this 50-mile mountain range is by taking the Motor Mountaineering Tour of Massanutten Mountain that Forest Service personnel have laid out. A descriptive brochure available at the Lee Ranger District Office in Edinburg, Virginia, offers points of interest from Camp Roosevelt south along Crisman Hollow Road and onto Elizabeth Furnace at

## :: Ratings

BEAUTY: ★ ★ ★
SITE PRIVACY: ★ ★ ★ ★
SPACIOUSNESS: ★ ★ ★ ★
QUIET: ★ ★ ★
SECURITY: ★ ★ ★
CLEANLINESS: ★ ★ ★

## :: Key Information

**ADDRESS:** Lee Ranger District, 102 Koontz Street, Edinburg, VA 22824

**OPERATED BY:** U.S. Forest Service

**CONTACT:** 540-984-4101; www.fs.usda.gov/gwj

**OPEN:** Beginning of May–end of September

**SITES:** 10

**SITE AMENITIES:** Picnic table, lantern pole, fire ring

**ASSIGNMENT:** First come, first served

**REGISTRATION:** Self-registration on site

**FACILITIES:** Water and flush toilets; no showers

**PARKING:** At campsites and in picnic area

**FEE:** $10 per night

**ELEVATION:** 1,200 feet

**RESTRICTIONS:**
- **Pets:** Must be on a leash no longer than 6 feet or under physical control at all times
- **Fires:** Use camp stoves and fire rings
- **Alcohol:** No restriction on responsible use
- **Vehicles:** No limit
- **Other:** Fires only in designated fire rings; campsites must be occupied the first night and attended for any subsequent period thereafter; no destruction of live trees

the northern end of Massanutten Mountain. Mountain bikers can pedal this tour.

Several well-blazed hiking trails geared toward both beginners and distance travelers run through this area. At the easier end of the spectrum are the paved 0.2-mile Discovery Way Trail and 0.5-mile Wildflower Trail, both of which are accessible from the Forest Service parking area on US 211 at the top of New Market Gap. Moving north, you'll find the 0.4-mile paved interpretive Massanutten Story, which offers signage to describe the vast geologic history of this mountain. At the end of the trail you'll enjoy some awesome views of neighboring Page County.

Mountain bikers and equestrians will find an extensive network of trails along Massanutten that can be pieced together with gravel Forest Service roads for a considerable number of routes. The 9-mile (point-to-point) Duncan Knob Hollow Trail is especially nice, as are the 2.1-mile Gap Creek and 2.8-mile Scothorn Gap Trails. The latter two connect Duncan Knob Hollow with Crisman Hollow, which has been carved out over time by Passage Creek. Anglers will enjoy going after the stocked trout in Passage Creek.

Camp Roosevelt is a great base from which to explore the beauty of the surrounding national forest. Additionally, nearby Luray features caverns, canoeing, and plenty of attractions for kids. Shenandoah Caverns and the New Market Battlefield, site of an 1864 Civil War battle in which 250 cadets from Virginia Military Institute successfully fought, are both nearby off of US 11, or you can go farther up into the mountains to explore Skyline Drive.

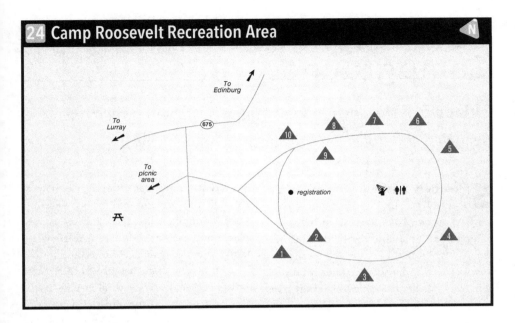

## 24 Camp Roosevelt Recreation Area

## :: Getting There

From I-81, take Exit 279. Turn east on VA 675. At the intersection of VA 675 and US 11 in the center of Edinburg, turn left onto US 11. At the north end of Edinburg, turn right and back onto VA 675. Follow SA 675 for 5.9 miles over Massanutten Mountain to the stop sign at Kings Crossing. Turn right and remain on VA 675 for 3.4 miles to the intersection of VA 675, FDR 274, and VA 730. Turn left and remain on VA 675 for 0.3 mile to the entrance to Camp Roosevelt on the left.

**GPS COORDINATES**   N38° 43.805  W78° 31.078

# 25

# Cave Mountain Lake Campground

*This area of the Shenandoah Valley is rife with limestone deposits, sinkholes, and the accompanying caves.*

**Splendidly nestled** at the foot of the peaks of the Blue Ridge Mountains is Cave Mountain Lake Recreation Area. The campground is a short walk through the woods away from the lake, which means that you won't get a view of the water from your tent flap. Fortunately, this separation gives campers some privacy from visitors who come for the day to swim in the 7-acre lake and eat at the adjoining picnic area.

The entrance road climbs and winds through a forest of pine, hemlock, and assorted hardwoods before dropping down into the wooded camping area. The sites are spread out along a large loop and small spur, with sites 36–38 designated as walk-in sites that offer a higher degree of privacy than the rest. All of the sites, however, are spacious, and the tall foliage creates privacy for each site. Tent pads consist of a fine gravel surface. The camping area features flush toilets, water hydrants, and showers. Sites 1–18, 20–27, 41, and 42 should be reserved

at **recreation.gov**. Back Run courses its way through the campground before entering Cave Mountain Lake. Back Run is usually placid and delightful but can overflow its banks after heavy rains. Plan accordingly.

Located a short distance from Natural Bridge Caverns and Natural Bridge itself, this area of the Shenandoah Valley is rife with limestone deposits, sinkholes, and the accompanying caves. The 90-foot Natural Bridge is an imposing limestone arch that stands 215 feet above the gorge carved out by Cedar Creek. Some consider it to be one of the seven natural wonders of the world. Certainly it is one of the wonders of the Shenandoah Valley. First discovered and worshipped as a sacred site by the Monocan Indians, Thomas Jefferson bought it in 1774 for 20 shillings from King George III. Jefferson envisioned it as "undoubtedly one of the sublimest curiosities in nature" and planned to make it open for the public to see. Rumor has it that if you look hard enough, you can even see the initials of a young George Washington carved into the side.

The other natural feature of the mountains bordering the Shenandoah Valley is the iron ore that the Confederacy depended on for munitions during the Civil War; the nearby Glenwood Iron Furnace was one of more than 100 in western Virginia that helped sustain the Southern cause. CCC workers who were camped at what was

## :: Ratings

BEAUTY: ★ ★ ★
SITE PRIVACY: ★ ★ ★ ★
SPACIOUSNESS: ★ ★ ★ ★
QUIET: ★ ★ ★
SECURITY: ★ ★ ★ ★
CLEANLINESS: ★ ★ ★ ★ ★

## :: Key Information

**ADDRESS:** Glenwood-Pedlar Ranger District, P.O. Box 10, Natural Bridge Station, VA 24579

**OPERATED BY:** U.S. Forest Service

**CONTACT:** 540-291-2188; www.fs.usda.gov/gwj

**OPEN:** April 1–Oct. 31

**SITES:** 41

**SITE AMENITIES:** Picnic table, fire grill, lantern pole

**ASSIGNMENT:** By reservation at www.fs.usda.gov/gwj

**REGISTRATION:** Self-registration on site

**FACILITIES:** Flush toilets, water, cold showers

**PARKING:** No more than 2 cars per site and confined to existing spurs and parking lots

**FEE:** $15 per night; includes access to beach

**ELEVATION:** 1,100 feet

**RESTRICTIONS:**

■ **Pets:** Must be on leash; prohibited on beach

■ **Fires:** In fireplaces only

■ **Alcohol:** Prohibited in beach area, parking lots, and picnic areas

■ **Vehicles:** Up to 30 feet on some sites

■ **Other:** No destruction of live trees; quiet time 10 p.m.–6 a.m.; firearms prohibited.

formerly the Natural Bridge Learning Center constructed the lake, built the dam, planted pines, and erected picnic structures at Cave Mountain Lake in the early 1930s. There's no shortage of natural and historic places to visit should you decide to use Cave Mountain Lake as a base camp from which to explore the area.

Both hikers and mountain bikers will enjoy the 4-mile Wildcat Mountain Trail, which takes off from the upper end of the campground and gains some 1,500 feet before looping back. Adventurous mountain bikers can pair this trail with one or more gravel forest development roads for even longer outings. Those looking for a shorter walk should try the 0.5-mile Panther Knob Nature Trail. Additional trails, including the famed Appalachian Trail, can be found in the James River Face Wilderness just 4 miles from the campground.

In addition to the wide, sandy lakeside beach, the day-use area includes a grassy field for tossing a ball around, a bathhouse, and 41 picnic sites. The rustic log pavilion was built by the CCC and can be reserved by groups of up to 50 people. Cave Mountain Lake is less than 10 miles from I-81, but its natural beauty and relative seclusion make it a worthwhile destination for those looking for solace.

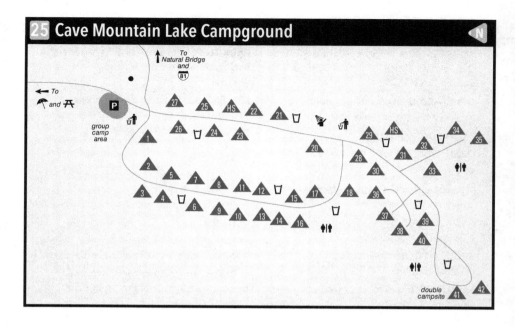

## :: Getting There

From I-81, take Exit 180 to US 11 to Natural Bridge. Follow VA 130 East from Natural Bridge 3 miles; then turn right onto VA 759. Follow VA 759 for 3.2 miles and turn right onto VA 781. Continue another 1.6 miles to the entrance for Cave Mountain Lake Recreation Area.

**GPS COORDINATES**   N37° 34.080  W79° 32.445

# 26

# Douthat State Park

*This CCC-constructed lakeside getaway in far-western
Virginia lies in a valley between Beards and Middle Mountains.*

**Scenic Douthat** State Park has been deemed one of the nation's top 10 state parks and honored with a Centennial Medallion from the American Society of Landscape Architects. These 4,493 acres were part of a land grant given to Robert Douthat by Governor Robert Brooke in 1795. In 1936, Douthat became one of the original six parks in the Virginia State Park system. This CCC-constructed lakeside getaway lies in a valley between Beards and Middle Mountains, through which Wilson Creek and VA 629 run. The neighboring peaks reach heights of 3,000 feet, while the lake is nestled at 1,146 feet.

The park's Depression-era beginnings led to its designation as a National Historic Landmark. Great fishing in the 50-acre lake, rental cabins, and more than 40 miles of hiking trails across the adjacent mountainsides are but a few of the attractions that draw large numbers of vacationers out to this rustic setting. Stone walls, log pavilions, and wrought-iron attachments all speak to the CCC craftsmanship. Another popular

stop is the recently renovated Lakeview Restaurant and Country Store.

Douthat's 87 campsites are divided among four campgrounds: Lakeside, White Oak, Beaver Dam, and Whispering Pines. Tent campers usually head for nonelectric Lakeside Campground, which is closest to the lake. The sites have no wooded privacy barriers, but the views of the lake and neighboring mountains are worth the compromise. Lakeside Campground is located between Beaver Dam Campground to the north and White Oak Campground to the south. Its 19 sites are accessible from VA 629 and are the most popular because of the outstanding views.

White Oak Campground is more RV oriented, but the entire area lies under the shade of towering hemlocks with varying degrees of separation from each other. White Oak is south of the beach, located by the contact station. While all 31 sites are wooded and private, those sites numbered in the 20s are especially desirable.

Equestrians have their own space with the 14-site Beaver Dam Equestrian Campground, which includes 12-foot-square stalls, electric and water hookups, and a dump station.

The 23-site Whispering Pines Campground is located approximately 3 miles south of the main park itself and officially became part of Douthat State Park in April of 2012. It is bordered by Wilson Creek, has

## :: Ratings

BEAUTY: ★ ★ ★ ★
SITE PRIVACY: ★ ★ ★
SPACIOUSNESS: ★ ★ ★
QUIET: ★ ★ ★
SECURITY: ★ ★ ★
CLEANLINESS: ★ ★ ★ ★

# :: Key Information

**ADDRESS:** 14239 Douthat State Park Road, Millboro, VA 24460

**OPERATED BY:** Virginia Department of Conservation and Recreation

**CONTACT:** 540-862-8100; virginiastateparks.gov

**OPEN:** First weekend in March–Dec. 1; water at campsites may not be available in late autumn due to freezing temperatures

**SITES:** 87

**SITE AMENITIES:** Picnic table, lantern pole, fire grill

**ASSIGNMENT:** First come, first served

**REGISTRATION:** Call 800-933-PARK or visit reserveamerica.com; site assignment on arrival

**FACILITIES:** Cabin and lodge rental; lake swimming, boating, and fishing; equestrian trails; flush toilets; hot showers; drink machine

**PARKING:** 2 vehicles per campsite in addition to camping unit; overflow parking available.

**FEE:** Standard lakeside sites (with electric but no water hookups), $26 per night; sites with electric and water hookups, $30 per night

**ELEVATION:** 1,367 feet

**RESTRICTIONS:**

▨ **Pets:** $5 per pet; attended, on 6-foot leash or shorter; not allowed in swimming areas or restrooms

▨ **Fires:** In fire rings, stoves, or grills only; do not bring firewood into park

▨ **Alcohol:** Prohibited

▨ **Vehicles:** 2 per site

▨ **Other:** Swimming is allowed in the designated beach area only; maximum stay is 14 days in a 30-day period; maximum 6 people or 1 family per site; quiet hours 10 p.m.–8 a.m.

its own lake for swimming, and includes water and electric hookups for RVs up to 50 feet long.

Those looking to minimally rough it should plan ahead and rent one of the park's 30 cabins, 25 of which were constructed from logs by CCC workers.

Besides the rustic natural setting, the park's main attraction is the lake, which is regularly stocked with trout. Fish from the shore; bring your own non-gasoline-powered boat; or rent a canoe, paddleboat, hydrobike, or "funyak" (available from the beginning of April through Labor Day). The 150-yard sandy beach is a great place to lounge, while the nearby two-story concession building offers restrooms, showers, and food.

There's no shortage of things to do here, so once you've pitched your tent, you can enjoy the area on foot, by bike, or by boat.

There's a considerable degree of exploring to be done in the neighboring national forest area, but Douthat State Park is a destination in and of itself.

The park's literature lists two dozen trails suitable for hiking and mountain biking. The 4.5-mile Stony Run Trail is Douthat's longest, although there are infinite possibilities for extending shorter trails into longer, more challenging outings. Douthat is rapidly gaining a following among recreational and competitive mountain bikers for the quality of the trails that traverse Middle Mountain, which rises to more than 3,000 feet on the western side of the park. Bikers flock to the park in May for the Middle Mountain Momma bike race. Race promoter Kyle Inman refers to Douthat as "mountain-bike Disneyland."

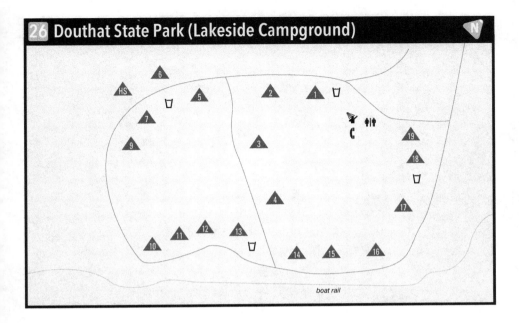

# 26 Douthat State Park (Lakeside Campground)

## :: Getting There

From I-64, take Exit 27 onto VA 629. Follow this road 3 miles to enter the park. The park office is 2 miles farther.

**GPS COORDINATES**    Lakeside Campground: N37° 54.597  W79° 47.839

Beaver Dam Campground: N37° 54.852  W79° 47.829

White Oak Campground: N37° 53.733  W79° 48.243

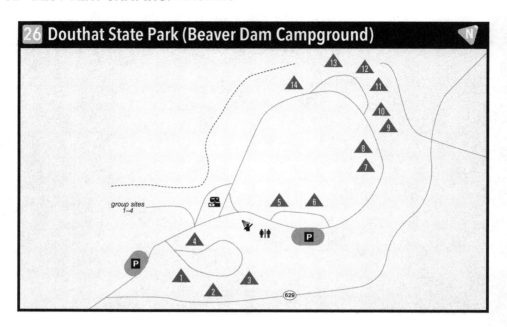

**26 Douthat State Park (Beaver Dam Campground)**

group sites
1–4

629

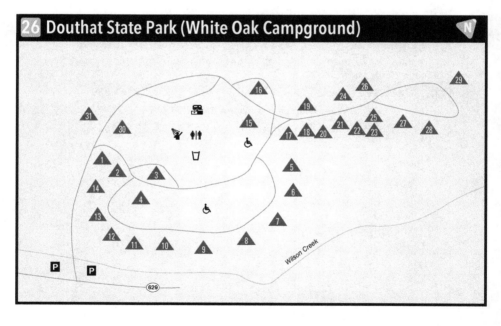

**26 Douthat State Park (White Oak Campground)**

Wilson Creek

629

# 27

# Elizabeth Furnace Recreation Area

*Fort Valley's natural camouflage has protected its inhabitants from development.*

**The Elizabeth Furnace Recreation Area** is nestled in Fort Valley, a 22-mile-long valley hidden at the northern end of the 50-mile-long Massanutten Mountain. You can easily drive right by Fort Valley without noticing it's there, and its elusiveness and inaccessibility have been exploited throughout history. In the 1700s, an English miner named Powell counterfeited coins from Fort Valley's ore and vanished into Fort Valley any time authorities tried to capture him. The locals referred to the area as Powell's Fort Valley. George Washington is said to have considered it both as an alternative to the winter camp at Valley Forge and as a last-resort bunker if things had gone badly during the Revolutionary War.

Fort Valley's natural camouflage has protected its inhabitants not just from invading armies but also from development. You won't find a Walmart or McDonald's in Fort Valley, and residents often must drive as much as 30 miles to get to a major supermarket. The valley is covered in undeveloped,

green national forest and farmland. Many of the original roads and trails were constructed by the Civilian Conservation Corps before World War II.

Today, Fort Valley is clearly marked on all Virginia maps, and VA 678 goes into the valley from Strasburg, so the campground is accessible from both urban Northern Virginia and Washington, D.C. The trails of Fort Valley and densely wooded campsites of Elizabeth Furnace get more than their share of use.

Access to this campground can be restricted after heavy rain, when the creek overflows its banks. Under average conditions, however, it provides a nice backdrop to this quiet campground, with waters that are stocked with trout for anglers. After passing the Volunteer Host site at the entrance to the campground, you'll find a large loop with some sites closer together than others; 9–17 are the more private settings. The campground is flat and forms a large loop around a grassy central area. A smaller loop near the campground entrance encompasses sites 24–30, but these are relatively close together. Water pumps and toilets are scattered about the campground. Showers and flush toilets are shut off in winter, but vault toilets operate year-round.

Virginia's Shenandoah Valley figures heavily into the country's history, especially during the Civil War. Iron ore was an

## :: Ratings

BEAUTY: ★ ★ ★
SITE PRIVACY: ★ ★ ★
SPACIOUSNESS: ★ ★ ★
QUIET: ★ ★ ★
SECURITY: ★ ★ ★
CLEANLINESS: ★ ★ ★

# :: Key Information

**ADDRESS:** Lee Ranger District, 102 Koontz Street, Edinburg, VA 22824

**OPERATED BY:** U.S. Forest Service

**CONTACT:** 540-984-4101; www.fs.usda.gov/gwj

**OPEN:** Year-round; running water during warm season only

**SITES:** 32

**SITE AMENITIES:** Fire ring, picnic table, lantern pole

**ASSIGNMENT:** First come, first served

**REGISTRATION:** Self-registration on site

**FACILITIES:** Water, hot showers, flush toilets, vault toilets

**PARKING:** At campsites, extra parking across VA 678; gates close to cars 9 p.m.–8 a.m.

**FEE:** $14 per night April–mid-October; $10 per night the rest of the year, when water is shut off in the bathhouse

**ELEVATION:** 770 feet

**RESTRICTIONS:**

▓ **Pets:** Must be on leash; clean up after pet

▓ **Fires:** Use camp stove or fire ring

▓ **Alcohol:** Prohibited in all campgrounds

▓ **Vehicles:** Up to 25 feet

▓ **Other:** Do not damage trees; quiet time 10 p.m.–6 a.m.; use tent pads; do not use faucets or sinks for fish, dishes, or personal items

early resource that was mined, purified in furnaces such as the one here at Elizabeth Furnace, and shipped by boat on the South Fork of the Shenandoah River to Hall Iron Works at Harpers Ferry, West Virginia. This iron was then used to make munitions for the Confederacy. Of the 14 furnaces in the state of Virginia in 1861, 8 similar furnaces were on what is now the Lee Ranger District. The 1830s log cabin at Elizabeth Furnace is open to the public on weekends as a Forest Service information center. Be sure to walk the Pig Iron (0.2-mile) and Charcoal (0.4-mile) Trails to learn more about this process.

Those looking for longer and more strenuous hikes can cross the road and climb on one or more of the area's well-blazed trails to Buzzard Rock Overlook, Fort Valley Overlook, or Signal Knob. From its strategic location at the northern end of the Shenandoah Valley—called the Lower Valley based on the

way the rivers flow through here—Signal Knob was an important Confederate lookout point to watch for the Union army in its attempt to enter and control the Shenandoah Valley. Massanutten Mountain trails are well marked and clear of blowdowns, thanks to the efforts of the Potomac Appalachian Trail Club. Mountain biking is also a possibility on these trails, but riders should be prepared to yield the right-of-way to hikers who frequent the area, especially on weekends.

The orange-blazed, 4.5-mile (point-to-point) Signal Knob Trail is a popular trail skirting the northern end of Massanutten and is part of the 71-mile Massanutten National Recreation Trail circling Fort Valley on what used to be known as the Massanutten East and West Trails. It offers some outstanding views, including those from Buzzard Rock Overlook and Fort Valley Overlook. To avoid a 9-mile out-and-back hike, plan to return via the

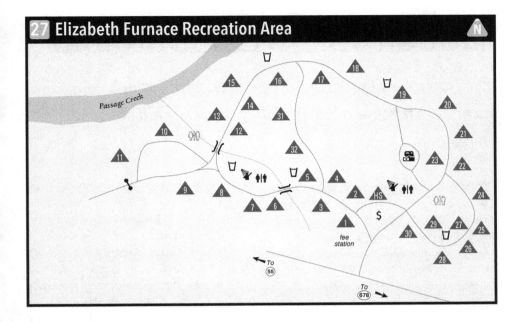

**27  Elizabeth Furnace Recreation Area**

Massanutten Mountain West and Bear Wallow Trails. A particularly picturesque spot is Mudhole Gap, through which Little Passage Creek passes between the Massanutten West Trail and FDR 66, Strasburg Reservoir Road.

Anglers will definitely want to bring their gear and do some fishing in the trout-stocked Passage Creek, which runs through this Recreation Area along VA 678. Fall-color season is also popular, when the leaves of Fort Valley take center stage.

## :: Getting There

From I-81, Exit 296, follow VA 55 east through Strasburg. Turn left at the traffic light in the middle of Strasburg, and remain on VA 55. Drive 5 miles before turning right onto VA 678 in the community of Waterlick. Go 3.5 miles to the campground entrance on the left.

**GPS COORDINATES**   N38° 55.470 W78° 19.926

# 28

# Hidden Valley Campground

*The floodplain bordering the Jackson River, which meanders through Hidden Valley, has very old stories to tell about this area.*

**T**ucked away in far-western Virginia at the base of Back Creek Mountain, Hidden Valley richly deserves its name. Looking out across the pasture adjacent to this wooded campground, moviegoers might recognize Warwickton, the antebellum mansion that provided the primary setting for the 1993 movie *Sommersby*, starring Jodie Foster and Richard Gere. Publicity releases said Hidden Valley was chosen as the location because "you could shoot 360 degrees and not know you were in the 20th century." Judge James Wood Warwick built the mansion in 1848, and it is considered one of the finest examples of Greek Revival architecture in western Virginia. It was placed on the National Register of Historic Places in 1973. When the Forest Service acquired it in 1965, the building was in a state of disrepair. The roof was replaced, but it wasn't until 1990 that new life was given to the structure. Pam and Ron Stidham of Ohio visited the area and ultimately entered into an agreement—the first of its kind in Forest Service

## :: Ratings

BEAUTY: ★ ★ ★ ★
SITE PRIVACY: ★ ★ ★
SPACIOUSNESS: ★ ★ ★
QUIET: ★ ★ ★
SECURITY: ★ ★ ★
CLEANLINESS: ★ ★ ★

history—to refurbish Warwickton and operate it with the Forest Service as the Hidden Valley Bed and Breakfast under a long-term special use permit.

The floodplain bordering the Jackson River, which meanders through Hidden Valley, has even older stories to tell about this area. Ongoing archaeological excavations have uncovered artifacts indicating the presence of American Indians dating back as early as 6500 B.C.

Hidden Valley Campground is located in a scenic, level setting and offers wooded serenity, provided you plan your visit outside of the November deer season. Although Virginia's Department of Game and Inland Fisheries went to a year-round trout season several years back, there's still a contingent of anglers who make their way to this stretch of the Jackson River in early spring out of habit. Almost any other time of year, however, you're likely to have your choice of campsites and few neighbors. The campground's 30 sites are shaded and set along a single loop. Vegetation between the large campsites provides a considerable amount of privacy.

The Jackson River is an excellent trout stream and is accessible via the Hidden Valley Trail, which starts at the mansion and follows the river for 5 miles—including several stream crossings sans bridges. This trail is also the start of a popular 12-mile mountain

# :: Key Information

**ADDRESS:** Warm Springs Ranger District, 422 Forestry Road, Hot Springs, VA 24445

**OPERATED BY:** U.S. Forest Service

**CONTACT:** 540-839-2521; www.fs.usda.gov/gwj

**OPEN:** Mid-March–end of November

**SITES:** 30

**SITE AMENITIES:** Picnic table, fire grill, lantern pole

**ASSIGNMENT:** First come, first served; no reservations

**REGISTRATION:** Self-registration on site

**FACILITIES:** Water and vault toilet

**PARKING:** At campsite

**FEE:** $10 per night

**ELEVATION:** 1,800 feet

**RESTRICTIONS:**
- **Pets:** On leash only
- **Fires:** In fire rings, stoves, or grills only
- **Alcohol:** May be consumed responsibly at campsite
- **Vehicles:** 25-foot limit
- **Other:** Do not carve, chop, or damage any live trees; keep noise at a reasonable level; maximum stay is 21 days in 30-day period; quiet time 10 p.m.–6 a.m.

bike loop that circles back on FDR 241-2 past the mansion. Other trails include the 0.6-mile Lower Lost Woman Trail and the 1-mile Upper Lost Woman Trail, both accessible from the campground. Other trails include River Loop, Cobbler Mountain, Muddy Run, Bogan Run, and Jackson River Gorge.

The Warm Springs Ranger District is a beautiful part of Virginia, and although you can have a dandy time exploring Hidden Valley without getting back into your car, plan to explore the Warm Springs/Hot Springs area. No visit would be complete without a healthy dip into Warm Springs, located at the intersection of VA 220 and VA 39. There are separate facilities for men and women, with the women's structure dating to 1836 and the men's to 1761, making it one of the oldest spas in the country. Indigenous people are thought to have frequented these springs as far back as 9,000 years ago.

Western Virginia was once famous for its healing springs, and wealthy urbanites spent their summers allowing the waters to cure what ailed them—as well as to escape mosquito-borne diseases and socialize at the resorts. Hot Springs was initially developed by early settlers Thomas Bullet and brothers Thomas and Andrew Lewis in 1766. This majestic resort is one of the few still in operation and has hosted many notables over the years, including Thomas Jefferson, Robert E. Lee, and J. P. Morgan. Jefferson said of the springs in *Notes on the State of Virginia:*

"They relieve rheumatisms. Other complaints also of very different natures have been removed or lessened by them . . . These springs are very much resorted to in spite of a total want of accommodation for the sick. Their waters are strongest in the hottest months, which occasions their being visited in July and August principally."

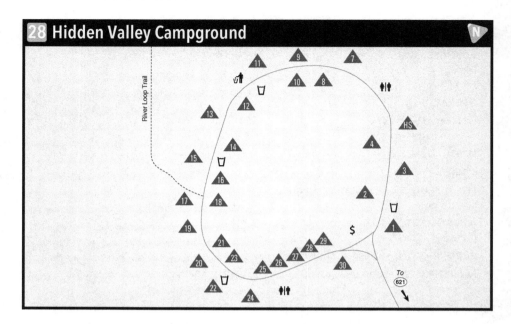

## :: Getting There

From Warm Springs, follow VA 39 west 3 miles. Turn right onto VA 621 and continue 1 mile. Turn left at the campground sign onto FDR 241, and proceed 1.5 miles to the entrance of Hidden Valley Campground.

**GPS COORDINATES**   N38° 05.925  W79° 49.305

# 29

# Hone Quarry Recreation Area

*If you're willing to camp with minimal facilities, you can enjoy pitching your tent throughout the year.*

The Hone Quarry Recreation Area lies at the foot of the Shenandoah Mountain on the western edge of the Shenandoah Valley. It's west of the city of Harrisonburg near the charming Briery Branch community along VA 257. Pull off the paved road onto Forest Road 62 after passing the Hone Quarry picnic area, and you'll arrive at the single loop containing the campground's 10 sites. The picnic area is popular among Rockingham County residents, but there are 23 grills and picnic tables, so you won't have trouble finding a spot during the week. The campground is set among mature hemlocks with campsites separated by an understory of young evergreens. The thick vegetation and minimal number of sites means you're likely to have ample privacy at Hone Quarry. Campers will find optimal seclusion during the week and outside of the busy summer months. The campground is a popular site for deer hunters in November, however, so plan

accordingly. If you're willing to camp with minimal facilities, you can enjoy pitching your tent throughout the year.

The trout-stocked Hone Quarry Run borders the campground, but like many mountain runoffs, this benign stream can overflow its banks quickly after heavy rains, flooding low-lying campsites. So it's best to avoid this area after wet weather. On the other hand, the stream tends to dry up in the summer. Somewhere in between you'll be lulled to sleep by the water's burble as it courses toward the North River.

The quarry itself is a popular fishing destination and is located past the campground on FDR 62. Swimming is prohibited. For alternate fishing destinations, Hearthstone Lake is just 7 miles away on FDR 101, and Switzer Lake is just north of here in the shadow of High Knob on US 33. For those who enjoy their trout fishing from closer banks, Hone Quarry Run is an option, as is Briery Branch Lake. Those looking to take a swim in the national forest will find Todd Lake Recreation Area, some 12.5 miles south of Hone Quarry, to be an inviting destination.

For spectacular views into West Virginia and across the Shenandoah Valley, leave the campground and turn right onto VA 924. Keep climbing Shenandoah Mountain until you reach the crest of Reddish

## :: Ratings

BEAUTY: ★ ★ ★
SITE PRIVACY: ★ ★ ★
SPACIOUSNESS: ★ ★ ★
QUIET: ★ ★
SECURITY: ★ ★ ★
CLEANLINESS: ★ ★ ★ ★

# :: Key Information

**ADDRESS:** North River Ranger District, 401 Oakwood Drive, Harrisonburg, VA 22801

**OPERATED BY:** U.S. Forest Service

**CONTACT:** 540-432-0187; www.fs.usda.gov/gwj

**OPEN:** Year-round; snow and ice may restrict winter use

**SITES:** 10

**SITE AMENITIES:** Fireplace grill, picnic table, lantern pole

**ASSIGNMENT:** Camper can choose from available sites

**REGISTRATION:** On arrival

**FACILITIES:** Vault toilets, well with hand pump

**PARKING:** At campsite and picnic area

**FEE:** $5 per night

**ELEVATION:** 1,880 feet

**RESTRICTIONS:**

■ **Pets:** On leash only

■ **Fires:** In fire rings, stoves, or grills only

■ **Alcohol:** Prohibited

■ **Vehicles:** Up to 21 feet

■ **Other:** Do not carve, chop, or damage any live trees; keep noise at a reasonable level; only non-gasoline-powered boats allowed in quarry; quiet time 10 p.m.–6 a.m.

---

Knob. Don't be surprised if you see some intrepid bicyclists attempting the assault on Reddish Knob. You'll find parking as well as an incredible panorama from this 4,397-foot perch. I was parked here one time enjoying the views when a fellow unloaded gear from his car. Minutes later he strapped a set of wings onto his back and launched himself into the air, becoming a soaring speck within a short time.

This section of the national forest is popular among Harrisonburg's large number of mountain bikers, and many of the more desirable trails and woods roads funnel down from Shenandoah Mountain and converge on Hone Quarry. Mud Pond Gap, Slate Springs Trail, and California Ridge are but a few of the local, well-used trails within a short distance of the Hone Quarry campground. This is a

great area for hikers and equestrians, but be prepared to share the trail whether you're on two legs or two wheels.

FDR 62 becomes increasingly rocky as it climbs Shenandoah Mountain toward Flagpole Knob. Along the way, the rough road ends where Mines Run Trail begins before merging into the Slate Springs Trails. If you're planning to do any exploring up here, pick up a national forest map of the North River District. Hone Quarry is set among an incredible network of trails, and these inexpensive maps will give you an idea of the trails that surround your campsite. Undoubtedly, you'll find, as I have over the years, that what's on the map and what's in the great beyond do not necessarily match up. And that can be the adventure or the danger of any outing in the backcountry.

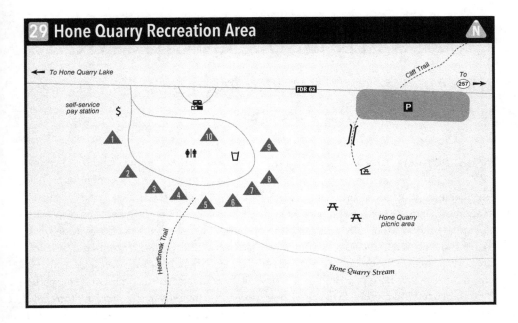

## :: Getting There

From Harrisonburg, take VA 42 south to Dayton. Turn right onto VA 257 and go west 11 miles before turning right onto FDR 62 and the entrance to Hone Quarry.

**GPS COORDINATES**  N38° 27.755  W79° 08.046

# 30

# Lake Robertson Campground

*Named for U.S. Senator A. Willis Robertson, this area is rife with history and natural beauty.*

The **581-acre** Lake Recreation Area lies at the western edge of the Shenandoah Valley at the foot of North Mountain. Early American Indians called this ridge Endless Mountain, and that's the image you'll get while looking up at it from the dam along the Lake Trail. An even better vantage point, however, is from North Mountain itself. Take a ride up to the mountain crest for an incredible panorama across Lexington and Rockbridge to the Blue Ridge Mountains.

From Lexington, it's a twisty but scenic route though Collierstown to Lake Robertson. After turning off VA 770 onto the park's entrance road, you may be surprised to find that this rural setting has playing fields; tennis, volleyball, and badminton courts; and a swimming pool. These facilities are in addition to the 26-acre fishing and boating lake. Rent a canoe or johnboat for a peaceful paddle, or cast a line at the bass, walleye, and sunfish that call Lake Robertson home.

There are also a number of short trails, from 0.25 mile to 1.75 miles, that circle the

## :: Ratings

BEAUTY: ★ ★ ★ ★
SITE PRIVACY:
SPACIOUSNESS: ★ ★ ★
QUIET: ★ ★ ★
SECURITY: ★ ★ ★ ★
CLEANLINESS: ★ ★ ★ ★

lake and continue uphill behind the campground. Those looking for more of a challenge can link the various trails together. Hikers and mountain bikers can also leave the park entirely and head for the wide-open spaces of the George Washington and Jefferson National Forests, which lie just west of here along North Mountain. The park's brochure includes a map showing the trails, which are also plainly marked in the wooded area west of the campground.

The campground is located behind the camp store and across the park's main drive from the lake. Situated in a grove of trees along a single loop, the sites have little privacy but ample shade from spring through summer. The campground slopes gently uphill with plenty of space between sites, especially those around the volleyball court at the top of the hill. Sites 26–30 surround the grassy hilltop and are a little farther from the park's other activities, while sites 20, 21, 23, and 25 are nearby along the edge of the campground road. Tent campers should be sure to bring a ground cloth and mattress pad because several of the tent pads are gravel.

Those familiar with Virginia politics may recognize the name of former U.S. Senator A. Willis Robertson, for whom this park is named. He was a Lexington resident and co-sponsored the Federal Aid in Wildlife Restoration Program, which has been credited with funneling billions of dollars to

## :: Key Information

**ADDRESS:** 106 Lake Robertson Drive, Lexington, VA 24450

**OPERATED BY:** Rockbridge County Parks and Recreation

**CONTACT:** 540-463-4164; www.co.rockbridge.va.us/departments /recreation/lake_robertson.htm

**OPEN:** April 1–end of November

**SITES:** 53

**SITE AMENITIES:** Picnic table, electric/ water hookups, fire ring

**ASSIGNMENT:** By reservation or on arrival

**REGISTRATION:** By reservation or on arrival

**FACILITIES:** Lake boating and fishing, swimming pool, playground, tennis courts, softball field, water, hot showers, flush toilets, camp store, pay phone, laundry, drink machines

**PARKING:** At campsites; max 2 vehicles

**FEE:** $26 per night for tent campers; $30 per night for trailers

**ELEVATION:** 1,540 feet

**RESTRICTIONS:**

■ **Pets:** Must be on leash, attended, and quiet at all times; pet-walking area; must clean up after pet

■ **Fires:** In camp stoves and fire rings only

■ **Alcohol:** Prohibited

■ **Vehicles:** No limit

■ **Other:** Maximum 6 people, 2 tents per site; no gas motors allowed

states for wildlife restoration work. Most of us are better acquainted with the senator's prominent son, evangelist and politician Pat Robertson. This area is, as mentioned, rife with history and natural beauty.

Surrounding Rockbridge County is named for Natural Bridge, a spectacular 215-foot-high arch eroded out of limestone by Cedar Creek. Plan to take a picnic lunch to nearby Goshen Pass, an awesome gorge where the Maury River has carved a path over time through the Allegheny Mountains. Lexington is the home of Washington and Lee University and the Virginia Military Institute. Stonewall Jackson owned a home here, and Civil War skirmishes were fought in the surrounding area.

You could use Lake Robertson campground as a base from which to explore the rich history and beauty of Rockbridge County and Lexington, located just 10 miles away. You could, however, just as easily park your car at Lake Robertson, pitch your tent, and savor the facilities that are provided. Either way, you're sure to enjoy your stay.

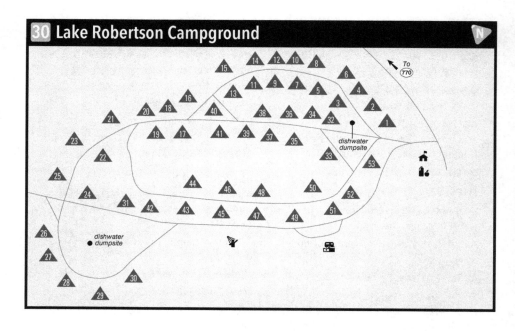

## :: Getting There

From Lexington, follow US 11 for a mile to VA 251. Stay on VA 251 for 10 miles to VA 770. Turn left and drive 2 miles to the park's entrance.

**GPS COORDINATES**   N37° 48.053  W79° 36.572

# 31

# Lewis Mountain Campground

*Here you'll find a quiet, rustic setting that is sometimes overlooked in favor of the park's larger campgrounds.*

**L**ewis **Mountain Campground** is located in the central section of Shenandoah National Park. With only 31 campsites, it's the smallest of the park's five campgrounds. Half are designated as tent sites and half for RVs. There are no electric hookups, and this is the only campground in Shenandoah National Park that does not have sewage disposal tanks. If you're fortunate enough to snag a site at Lewis Mountain, you'll find a quiet, rustic setting that is sometimes overlooked in favor of the larger campgrounds.

After pulling off Skyline Drive at milepost 57.5, you'll first pass through the Lewis Mountain picnic area and then pass rental cabins before reaching the campground. The campground consists of one large loop with two smaller loops carved out among mature maple, pine, hemlock, and oak trees, with little vegetation to screen one campsite from another. Of the 31 sites, 11, 14, 15, 16, and 18 are the more private. The tent pads are gravel, so a ground cloth and sleeping pad are highly recommended. It is not possible to reserve a site in advance, so at the busiest times, like autumn weekends, you won't be able to drive in and find a site. As with the other Shenandoah National Park campgrounds, it's best to plan your arrival during the week, especially if you're coming to see the spectacular October leaves. Be sure to pick up a copy of *Explore Shenandoah*, the park's newsletter, for a great overview of where things are located in Shenandoah National Park, as well as times and locations for ranger programs.

At the campground, you'll be welcomed by a sign that reads "Bear Country—Protect Your Property and Food—Proper Food Storage Is Required." This is not an idle warning, and campers should use the food-storage facility in the campground. It's especially important not to eat or store food in your tent, lest you have unwanted late-night visitors of the large and furry kind.

This campground doesn't offer access to an abundance of hiking trails as do the park's other campgrounds. However, nowhere in Shenandoah National Park are you too far from the more than 500 miles of trails that crisscross the 196,000-acre park. The half-mile (point-to-point) Lewis Mountain East Trail departs from site 16 on its short ascent to Lewis Mountain via a mossy and fern-lined path. Numerous other hikes are accessible via the Appalachian Trail, which you can reach from site 3. Just as the 105-mile Skyline Drive forms the park's

## :: Ratings

BEAUTY: ★ ★ ★ ★
SITE PRIVACY: ★ ★ ★
SPACIOUSNESS: ★ ★ ★
QUIET: ★ ★ ★ ★
SECURITY: ★ ★ ★ ★
CLEANLINESS: ★ ★ ★ ★ ★

## :: Key Information

**ADDRESS:** Skyline Drive, milepost 57.5

**OPERATED BY:** National Park Service

**CONTACT:** 540-999-3500, ext. 3231; nps.gov/shen

**OPEN:** Weather dependent; early spring–late autumn

**SITES:** 31

**SITE AMENITIES:** Picnic table, fire grill

**ASSIGNMENT:** Campers can choose from available sites

**REGISTRATION:** On arrival

**FACILITIES:** Camp store, laundry, coin-operated showers, flush toilets

**PARKING:** At campsite and next to camp store

**FEE:** $15 per night in addition to $15 park entrance fee; discounts for holders of Interagency Senior/Access passes and Golden Age/Access passes

**ELEVATION:** 3,396 feet

**RESTRICTIONS:**

■ **Pets:** Must be attended and on leash shorter than 6 feet; clean up after pet

■ **Fires:** Only in camp stoves and fireplaces; downed wood can be collected, but firewood cannot be brought into the park

■ **Alcohol:** Permitted

■ **Vehicles:** Up to 30 feet on pull-through sites

■ **Other:** Do not damage any trees; wash dishes at campsite, not at restrooms (but gray water must be disposed of in service sinks at restrooms); maximum 6 people, 2 tents, 2 vehicles per site; quiet hours 10 p.m.–6 a.m.; noise limit for generators and use restricted to 8–10 a.m. and 4–7 p.m.

backbone for driving, 101 miles of the Appalachian Trail form a spine of sorts for hikers. Shenandoah's abundant side trails are just a short drive away.

Either by walking south along the Appalachian Trail or driving on Skyline Drive to milepost 59.5, you can reach the start of the Pocosin Mission Trail. You'll pass one of the Potomac Appalachian Trail Cabins as you amble along the fire road to the site of an old Episcopal mission established around 1904, complete with a fascinating, overgrown cemetery. Turn around and head back for a pretty, easy 1.9-mile walk in the woods. Stretch this into a longer and more challenging 5.6-mile out-and-back by continuing on

the yellow-blazed trail to Pocosin Hollow before returning.

Head north a short distance to milepost 56.4 to get onto the Bearfence Mountain Trail. You'll do your share of huffing and puffing as you scramble over the volcanic boulders, but by the time you reach the 3,640-foot summit of Bearfence Mountain, you'll enjoy a panoramic view that on a clear day will seem to go on forever. Backtrack or loop around for a 1.2-mile outing. Be sure to pick up one of the trail guides to Shenandoah Park that are listed in the Appendix for a more complete selection of places to walk in the vicinity of Lewis Mountain Campground.

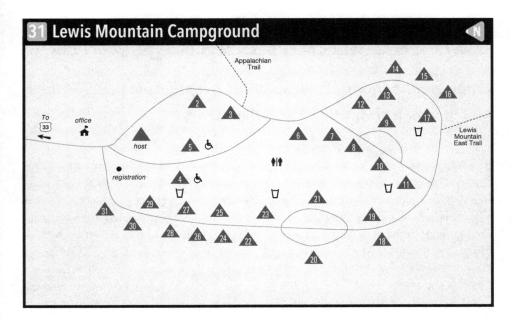

## :: Getting There

From the Swift Run Gap Entrance Station at mile 65.7 and US 33, drive north on Skyline Drive to the campground entrance at mile 57.5.

**GPS COORDINATES**   N38° 26.187  W78° 28.672

# 32

# Loft Mountain Campground

*Enjoy great panoramic views of the neighboring peaks, valley, and piedmont from this 3,400-foot perch.*

**L**oft Mountain Campground is located just off Skyline Drive in the southern section of Shenandoah National Park at mile 79.5. It is unique among the park's other campgrounds in that it is located at the top of Big Flat Mountain. As a result, there are great east and west panoramic views of the neighboring peaks, valley, and piedmont from this 3,400-foot perch. Another unusual feature at Loft Mountain Campground is the absence of mature, lofty hardwood trees that populate most of Shenandoah National Park. This mountaintop was once pastureland, so instead of trees there is an abundance of thick, low-growing shrubbery. This offers a considerable degree of privacy between campsites, and the dense vegetation diminishes the feeling of being crowded at Skyline Drive's largest campground, which contains 201 sites. Loft Mountain Campground is the southernmost of Shenandoah's campgrounds and is the ideal base from which to explore this end of the national park.

Loop A circumscribes the entire campground, with smaller loops B–G cutting across the center of loop A. Most of the sites are private and spacious, but those who want to completely avoid RVs and enjoy the feeling of being off by themselves should look at the 54 walk-in tent sites located on the outer edge of loop A. Parking is nearby, with one space reserved for each site, but you'll have to carry your gear a short distance to your home in the woods, which includes a picnic table, grill, and tent area.

Fall weekends are the most popular times for camping here, as well as in the rest of Shenandoah National Park, and sites are available on a first-come, first-serve basis. Reservations are not accepted at Loft Mountain Campground; only Big Meadows sites can be reserved. Signs at the entrances to Shenandoah National Park indicate site availability; if no sites are available, you can drive down the mountain to one of the private campgrounds outside the park in the Shenandoah Valley. Arrive during the week if you wish to have your choice of places to pitch your tent in one of Shenandoah National Park's developed campgrounds. On one balmy October weekend, the only available site I saw was roped off and set up with a bear trap. Take National Park Service warnings about bears seriously, unless you want unwelcome visitors during the night. Use bear-proof food-storage devices or lock

## :: Ratings

BEAUTY: ★ ★ ★ ★
SITE PRIVACY: ★ ★ ★ ★
SPACIOUSNESS: ★ ★ ★ ★
QUIET: ★ ★ ★ ★
SECURITY: ★ ★ ★ ★
CLEANLINESS: ★ ★ ★ ★ ★

# :: Key Information

**ADDRESS:** Skyline Drive, milepost 79.5

**OPERATED BY:** National Park Service

**CONTACT:** 540-999-3500, ext. 3231; nps.gov/shen

**OPEN:** Weather dependent; early spring–late autumn

**SITES:** 201

**SITE AMENITIES:** Picnic table, fire grill

**ASSIGNMENT:** First come, first served

**REGISTRATION:** On arrival

**FACILITIES:** Camp store, laundry, coin-operated showers, restaurant, flush toilets

**PARKING:** At campsite and limited parking beyond site A40 near exit

**FEE:** $15 per night, plus $15 park entrance fee

**ELEVATION:** 3,400 feet

**RESTRICTIONS:**

■ **Pets:** On 6-foot leash or shorter; clean up after pet

■ **Fires:** In camp stoves and designated fireplaces only; deadwood may be gathered but not brought into the park

■ **Alcohol:** Permitted

■ **Vehicles:** Up to 30 feet

■ **Other:** Do not damage any trees; wash dishes at campsite; discard gray water in restroom service sinks; quiet hours 10 p.m.–6 a.m.; maximum 6 people, 2 tents, 2 vehicles per site

your food away in your car trunk, and never keep food in your tent.

The Loft Mountain Information Center and Loft Mountain Amphitheater feature ranger programs, including campfires, guided walks, talks, and junior ranger programs for kids. There is no shortage of hiking trails near the campground and the southern section of the park. The Appalachian Trail loops around the southern end of the campground, leading off from sites A32 and A8. Additionally, numerous trails and two waterfalls at Doyles River Falls are close to the campground. Be sure to pick up a copy of *Explore Shenandoah,* the park's newsletter, for a great overview of where things are located in Shenandoah National Park, as well as times and locations for ranger programs.

One of the more popular side trails is the 1.3-mile Deadening Nature Trail loop. There are two rocky observation points that offer breathtaking views of the surrounding mountains and valleys. For a longer version of this hike, follow the Appalachian Trail north from the campground for 1.2 miles to create a 3.7-mile loop. Another hike that's well worth the effort is the 2.7-mile Loft Mountain Loop, which uses other trails, as well as the Appalachian Trail, to extend the Deadening Trail a bit. It will take you to a 3,290-foot perch on the side of Loft Mountain for some equally awesome views. On a clear day, you can see west to Massanutten Mountain.

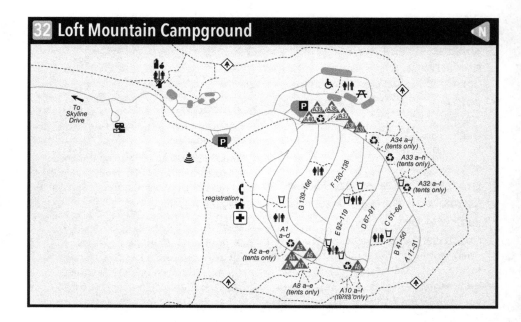

## :: Getting There

From the Swift Run Gap Entrance Station at mile 65.7, drive south on Skyline Drive to the campground entrance at milepost 79.5.

**GPS COORDINATES**  N38° 14.852  W78° 40.094

# 33

# Mathews Arm Campground

*Despite the uneven slope over much of Mathews Arm Campground, campsites are level; you'll have no trouble pitching your tent.*

**M**athews Arm is the northernmost campground in Shenandoah National Park. While it has flushing toilets, it is the only Skyline Drive campground without showers or a camp store. But don't let this discourage you from camping here. Fall-color October weekends and high-summer weekends are the busiest times in Shenandoah National Park. Sites can be difficult to come by, even though there are four campgrounds and 647 sites. Mathews Arm is often the last one to fill, but it is only 2 miles from Elkwallow Wayside's camping supplies and food service. Campers can use the coin-operated showers at any of the other campgrounds. These same campgrounds are almost empty during the week at the same times of year, but Mathews Arm, with its private, spacious walk-in tent sites, is deserving of consideration even when the other campgrounds are vacant. Despite the campground's elevation, cell phone coverage can be spotty.

Shenandoah National Park's 196,000 acres are closer to more people than any other National Park, and roughly 1.5 million get on the 105-mile Skyline Drive to visit the park every year. Skyline Drive and its sister road, the Blue Ridge Parkway, run along the top of the Blue Ridge Mountains. Skyline Drive can be accessed by entrances at Front Royal (mile 0), Thornton Gap (mile 31.5), Swift Run Gap (mile 65.7), and Rockfish Gap (mile 104.6). Mathews Arm Campground is easily accessed from Thornton Gap.

After pulling off Skyline Drive at mile 22.2, you'll descend to the Mathews Arm registration station. You'll pass the trailer dump station on the left and a parking area on the right, and will then enter the campground consisting of loops A, B, and C. Privacy is provided by mature oak and hickory trees, as well as the numerous rock outcrops that punctuate the area. Despite the uneven slope over much of Mathews Arm Campground, campsites are level; you'll have no trouble pitching your tent. Those sites closest to the entrance station are more open and will attract RVers, despite the lack of RV hookups. While there are many desirable sites throughout the campground, most are adjacent to one of the loop roads.

Opportunities for hiking abound, with 101 miles of the 2,100-mile Appalachian Trail running through the park. Many thru-hikers agree that the section of Appalachian Trail through Shenandoah National Park is the most beautiful of the

## :: Ratings

BEAUTY: ★ ★ ★ ★
SITE PRIVACY: ★ ★ ★ ★
SPACIOUSNESS: ★ ★ ★ ★
QUIET: ★ ★ ★ ★
SECURITY: ★ ★ ★ ★
CLEANLINESS: ★ ★ ★ ★ ★

## :: Key Information

**ADDRESS:** Skyline Drive, milepost 22.2

**OPERATED BY:** National Park Service

**CONTACT:** 540-999-3132; nps.gov/shen

**OPEN:** Weather dependent; spring–October

**SITES:** 178

**SITE AMENITIES:** Picnic table and fire grill

**ASSIGNMENT:** First come, first served; reserve at recreation.gov or 877-444-6777

**REGISTRATION:** On arrival

**FACILITIES:** Flush toilets

**PARKING:** At campsite and near amphitheater

**FEE:** $15 per night, plus $15 park entrance fee; discounts for holders of Interagency Senior/Access passes and Golden Age/Access passes

**ELEVATION:** 2,800 feet

**RESTRICTIONS:**

■ **Pets:** Must be attended and on leash shorter than 6 feet; clean up after pet

■ **Fires:** Only in camp stoves and fireplaces; firewood cannot be brought into park; use of downed wood is allowed

■ **Alcohol:** Permitted

■ **Vehicles:** No limit

■ **Other:** Do not carve, chop, or damage any standing trees; wash dishes at campsite, not at restrooms (but gray water must be disposed of in service sinks at restrooms); maximum 6 people, 2 tents, 2 vehicles per site; quiet hours 10 p.m.–6 a.m.; noise limit for generators and use restricted to 8–10 a.m. and 4–7 p.m.

trail's entire length from Georgia to Maine. Shenandoah also includes more than 400 additional miles of trails, most of which connect to the Appalachian Trail. Bicycling is popular on paved Skyline Drive, but bikes are prohibited on trails within the park. Be sure to pick up a copy of *Explore Shenandoah,* the park's newsletter, for a great overview of where things are located in Shenandoah National Park, as well as times and locations for ranger programs.

A population of some 6,000 white-tailed deer resides within the park's boundaries, and you're sure to encounter them at some time during your visit. Keep in mind, however, that it is illegal to feed park animals. An estimated 300–600 black bears also live in Shenandoah National Park. Seriously heed park warnings about bears: Keep food out of your tent and at least 100 yards away, and

use park-provided, bear-proof food-storage devices or suspend food from trees at least 10 feet from the ground and 4 feet from either tree. The tents-only area at Mathews Arm Campground features several food-storage devices. Several pleasant trails can be accessed from the campground. The 1.7-mile Traces Nature Trail is a mostly level loop that starts from the parking area by the registration station and circles Mathews Arm Campground. It also connects with the Mathews Arm Trail, a gated service road that starts at the end of the tents-only section. The trail proceeds downhill before intersecting with the Tuscarora–Overall Run Trail that takes you down to the picturesque 93-foot Overall Run Falls after a roughly 2-mile walk. Staying on the entire 4.4-mile Mathews Arm Trail will lead you along Mathews Arm Ridge to the Shenandoah National Park boundary.

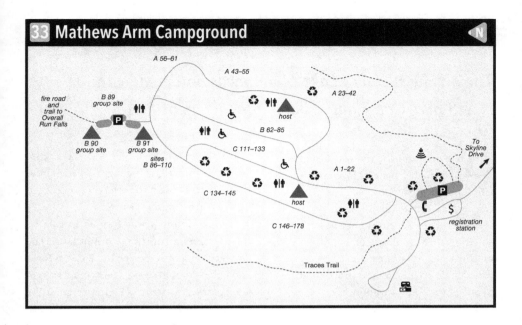

## 33 Mathews Arm Campground

## :: Getting There

From the Thornton Gap entrance (mile 31.5) to Shenandoah National Park, drive north on Skyline Drive to the entrance to Mathews Arm Campground at milepost 22.2.

**GPS COORDINATES**   N38° 45.605  W78° 17.867

# 34

# Morris Hill Campground

*The northern end of Lake Moomaw is bordered by the 13,428-acre Gathright Wildlife Management Area.*

**O**n a hilltop near the southern end of man-made Lake Moomaw, Morris Hill Campground features a loop of 39 non-reservable tent sites around a heavily wooded ravine. A nearby spur has 16 reservable sites that can house tents or RVs. Three of the reservable sites are categorized as wheelchair accessible and are located next to one of the three bathhouses.

All of the sites are situated in an area of mature hardwoods with enough low-growth vegetation to provide privacy between campsites. There is also ample space between campsites so that you won't feel that you're camping cheek by jowl. The central ravine adds significantly to the feeling of being nestled in the nearby George Washington National Forest.

A short walk via the Morris Hill Trail (0.75 mile point-to-point) or the Fortney Branch Trail (1.3 miles point-to-point) will take you to the lake. This 2,500-acre lake straddles the Alleghany–Bath county line, and recreational facilities are managed by two national forest ranger districts. The

## :: Ratings

BEAUTY: ★ ★ ★
SITE PRIVACY: ★ ★ ★ ★
SPACIOUSNESS: ★ ★ ★ ★
QUIET: ★ ★ ★
SECURITY: ★ ★ ★
CLEANLINESS: ★ ★ ★

southern end, where Morris Hill Campground is located, is managed by the James River District; the northern end is managed by the Warm Springs District.

Lake Moomaw was formed in 1981 by the construction of the Gathright Dam. The dam's cooling tower keeps the Jackson River and Lake Moomaw waters temperate even in late summer, giving the region some of the best trout fishing in Virginia. The area also supports abundant wildlife, including wild turkeys, white-tailed deer, and the occasional black bear. The average depth of the lake is 80 feet, its shoreline is 43.5 miles, and its length is 12 miles. It took two years to fill the lake. Surrounding the northern end of Lake Moomaw is the 13,428-acre Gathright Wildlife Management Area, one of the earliest tracts owned by Virginia's Department of Game and Inland Fisheries.

Anglers will find a number of fish, including largemouth bass, bluegill, crappie, and channel catfish. Fishing is allowed from the shore, the lake, and the dam, but not from the boat docks or beach. Boats can be launched from Fortney Branch and Coles Point, but boat lengths are restricted to 25 feet or less. Coles Point also features 20 picnic tables, two reservable picnic shelters, a bathhouse, and a half-acre sandy beach where swimmers and sunbathers can enjoy the southern end of Lake Moomaw. Swimming is not recommended in other parts of the south end of the lake.

## :: Key Information

**ADDRESS:** James River Ranger District, 810-A Madison Avenue, Covington, VA 24426

**OPERATED BY:** U.S. Forest Service

**CONTACT:** 540-962-2214; www.fs.usda.gov/gwj

**OPEN:** April 30–Nov. 1

**SITES:** 55

**SITE AMENITIES:** Picnic table, fire ring

**ASSIGNMENT:** Reserve at recreation.gov or 877-444-6777, or on arrival

**REGISTRATION:** Self-registration on site

**FACILITIES:** Lake swimming, boating, and fishing; flush toilets; hot showers

**PARKING:** Only on campsite spur

**FEE:** $18 per night

**ELEVATION:** 2,000 feet

**RESTRICTIONS:**
■ **Pets:** Must be on leash and attended

■ **Fires:** Only in fire rings and camp stoves

■ **Alcohol:** May be consumed responsibly at campsite

■ **Vehicles:** Some sites will handle any size RV

■ **Other:** Quiet time 10 p.m.–6 a.m.; campsite should be attended within 24-hour period

In addition to the Fortney Branch and Morris Hill Trails, which are accessible from the campground, 5.3-mile (point-to-point) Oliver Mountain Trail is a steep climb that offers breathtaking views of neighboring peaks and of the southern end of Lake Moomaw.

The Morris Hill Campground sits 18 miles north of Covington and I-64 along VA 605. It is a good place to hang your hat while touring Virginia's Western Highlands—formerly called the Alleghany Highlands; the name was changed to avoid confusion with the nearby Allegheny Mountains.

Morris Hill Campground should be considered to be just the tip of Lake Moomaw's amazing iceberg, as there are several other national forest campgrounds at various points along the lake shoreline. Bolar Mountain Recreation Area lies on the northwest shore of Lake Moomaw and offers 122 single and double campsites along four loops. These sites hug the shoreline and offer some great views, but with electric hookups and a dump station, they are geared towards RVs. Farther upstream you'll find 21 single-family sites with vault toilets and a hand-pumped water source. For the ultimate in private stays under a canopy of nylon and a ceiling of stars, it is also permissible to pick out any beautiful spot in the George Washington and Jefferson National Forests to pitch a tent, as long as there are no signs indicating otherwise.

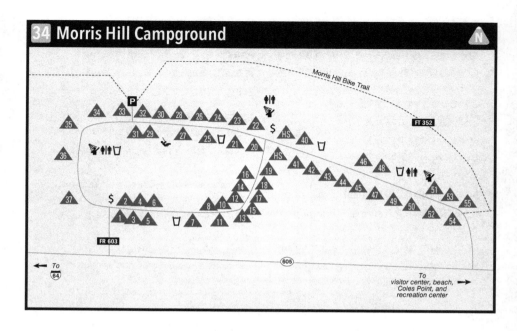

## :: Getting There

From I-64, take Exit 16 and follow US 220 north 4 miles. Turn left onto VA 687, and follow it 3 miles. Turn left onto VA 641, and go 1 mile before turning right onto VA 666. Continue 5 miles, and then turn right onto VA 605. You'll find FDR 603, the entrance to the Morris Hill Campground, 2 miles ahead.

**GPS COORDINATES** N37° 55.856 W79° 58.256

# 35

# North Creek Campground

*This no-frills area is shadowed by towering hemlocks and even more towering mountain ridges.*

**N**orth Creek Campground lies secluded at the foot of the Blue Ridge Mountains. It is a no-frills area where you can pitch a tent in the shadow of towering hemlocks and even more towering mountain ridges, with few other campers around. There is no bathhouse, just vault toilets and water pumps, but camping at North Creek is several steps above backpacking. You can drive to your site along a fast-moving trout stream and find a grill on which to cook your catch of the day or something from your cooler, with a picnic table on which to eat or just sit. Additionally, there is a garbage bin, dump station, and helpful volunteer campground host. North Creek Campground is not representative of all the campgrounds in this guide, but in many ways its scenic location and relatively primitive facilities connote the essence of what *Best Tent Camping* is all about. Not everyone is looking for this kind of back-to-nature experience, nor is it readily accessible to most people. And so this book contains a sampling of camping

experiences with a variety of amenities and, ideally, something for everybody.

The campground is bordered by North Creek, a stocked trout stream that completely encircles this spartan 15-site facility en route to the James River, which is located just west of here. All of these insular sites lie on a single gravel loop along the creek in an area of dense pine and hemlock trees with understory vegetation that allows for separation between sites. The better-than-average size of the sites, combined with the privacy from others, means that campers are likely to find ample seclusion here. Sites 6 and 7 are designated as a double site for larger parties. All others are singles.

Visitors should keep in mind that in spite of the beautiful setting, mountain run-offs like North Creek are quite susceptible to flooding after heavy rains. Plan and respond accordingly. In addition, the campground and FDR 59 are situated in a narrow valley between neighboring ridges, so the possibility for flash flooding is increased. Traces of past high water may be readily apparent.

Activities at the North Creek Campground all take advantage of this rich natural setting. Trout fishing from your tent site or somewhere downstream is an obvious choice if you wish to test your angling abilities against stocked and native species. Fly-fishermen will enjoy the special regulation area upstream from the campground where only artificial lures can be used. Check state

## :: Ratings

BEAUTY: ★ ★ ★ ★
SITE PRIVACY: ★ ★ ★ ★
SPACIOUSNESS: ★ ★ ★
QUIET: ★ ★ ★
SECURITY: ★ ★
CLEANLINESS: ★ ★ ★

## :: Key Information

| | |
|---|---|
| **ADDRESS:** Glenwood-Pedlar Ranger District, P.O. Box 10, Natural Bridge Station, VA 24579 | **ELEVATION:** 1,200 feet |
| **OPERATED BY:** U.S. Forest Service | **RESTRICTIONS:** |
| **CONTACT:** 540-291-2188; www.fs.usda.gov/gwj | ■ **Pets:** Attended; on 6-foot leash or shorter |
| **OPEN:** March 15–early December | ■ **Fires:** Only in stoves, grills, and fire rings |
| **SITES:** 15 | ■ **Alcohol:** No restriction except in day-use area by the lake |
| **SITE AMENITIES:** Picnic table, fire ring, lantern pole | ■ **Vehicles:** Up to 22 feet |
| **ASSIGNMENT:** First come, first served | ■ **Other:** Do not damage trees; quiet hours 10 p.m.–6 a.m.; no fireworks; firearms permitted only during hunting seasons with license; firearms must be broken down and cased within campground; maximum 8 people, 2 tents, 2 vehicles per site; generators allowed to run a maximum of 2 hours per day |
| **REGISTRATION:** Self-registration on site | |
| **FACILITIES:** Vault toilet, water | |
| **PARKING:** At sites only | |
| **FEE:** $10 per night | |

regulations as to which specific licenses are required. Bear in mind that North Creek can get crowded during hunting season; consider other nearby campgrounds as backup sites.

There is no shortage of hiking and mountain biking opportunities here in the George Washington and Jefferson National Forests. An especially scenic walk is the 2-mile (point-to-point) moderate climb on the Apple Orchard Falls National Recreation Trail, located at the end of FDR 59. The trail is well maintained and graded as it follows North Creek up the Blue Ridge Mountains. After the falls, it's another mile to the famed Appalachian National Scenic Trail, which stretches 2,200 miles from Georgia to Maine. Mountain bikers will find even more opportunities to pedal through the area by tackling the 2.6-mile Whitetail Trail loop or heading out on neighboring forest development roads that loop across Pine, Thomas, and Wildcat Mountains. Another option is to ride across Hoop Hole Gap to Cave Mountain Lake, take a swim, and pedal back to North Creek.

Whether you come here for outdoor challenges or quiet respite, you're sure to get your batteries recharged after a few days at North Creek.

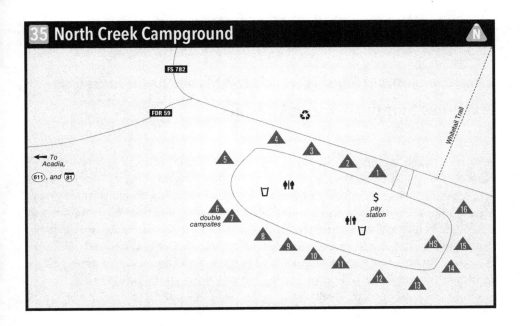

## :: Getting There

From I-81, take Exit 168 onto VA 614. Follow VA 614 for 3 miles before turning left onto FDR 59. Continue 2.5 miles to North Creek Campground.

**GPS COORDINATES**   N37° 32.531  W79° 35.007

# 36

# Otter Creek Campground

*This level campground is wooded with mountain laurel, oaks, and pines that provide ample shade.*

**O**tter Creek Campground lies near the lowest point (649 feet) on the Blue Ridge Parkway, whose 469 miles of two-lane blacktop are among the most spectacular in the country. Curiously, the highest point on the Virginia section of the parkway is only 15 miles south of here. This should give you an idea of the overall up-and-down nature of this famed scenic byway, which also has flat sections. The Blue Ridge Parkway begins numerically at milepost 0, located north of here at Afton Mountain, where Skyline Drive and the Blue Ridge Parkway meet.

Otter Creek Campground is situated at mile 60.9, north of the James River and US 501. The campground itself is located just behind the Otter Creek Restaurant and Gift Shop. After passing the entrance station and crossing Otter Creek, you'll find yourself at the center of a figure-eight road with smaller loop A for RVs on the left and loop B for tent campers on the right. Loop B is further bisected by a road that incorporates sites 41–45. The level campground is wooded with mountain laurel, oaks, and pines that

provide ample shade. The sites are well spaced, although parking spots for some sites are adjacent and the accompanying sites are relatively close together. If you want to fish for trout from your campsite or be lulled to sleep by the burble of Otter Creek, then plan to arrive during the week, when you can have your choice of creekside sites 1–9.

The 3.5-mile (one-way) Otter Creek Trail is a nice, relatively easy walk that runs from the restaurant parking lot to the James River Visitor Center, located just south of the campground along the James River. It crosses the creek twice before intersecting with the 0.9-mile Otter Lake Trail, which in turn loops around this small body of water.

The Otter Creek Campground works well as a base camp from which to explore the area or as a stopover on your way north or south. Plan to pack your bicycle, if for no other reason than just to ride the paved road that follows the undulations of the famed Blue Ridge Mountains. Paddling on the James, hiking on the Appalachian Trail that crosses US 501 just south of the campground, and mountain biking in the surrounding George Washington and Jefferson National Forests are all within a 15-minute drive. The Appalachian Trail and six others crisscross the 11,500-acre James River Face and adjoining Thunder Ridge wilderness areas just south of the James River. Nineteen miles of trails await mountain bikers at the South Pedlar ATV trail system, located

## :: Ratings

BEAUTY: ★ ★ ★
SITE PRIVACY: ★ ★ ★
SPACIOUSNESS: ★ ★ ★
QUIET: ★ ★ ★
SECURITY: ★ ★ ★
CLEANLINESS: ★ ★ ★

## :: Key Information

**ADDRESS:** Blue Ridge Parkway, 199 Hemphill Knob Road, Asheville, NC 28803

**OPERATED BY:** National Park Service

**CONTACT:** 434-299-5941; nps.gov/blri

**OPEN:** May 1–Oct. 31; occasional reduced-fee, reduced-service winter camping available

**SITES:** 45

**SITE AMENITIES:** Picnic table, fire ring, lantern pole

**ASSIGNMENT:** First come, first served

**REGISTRATION:** Self-registration on site

**FACILITIES:** Restaurant, water, flush toilets

**PARKING:** At campsites only

**FEE:** $14 per night (varies by season)

**ELEVATION:** 777 feet

**RESTRICTIONS:**

▓ **Pets:** Must be attended and on leash shorter than 6 feet; clean up after pet

▓ **Fires:** Use camp stoves and fireplaces; deadwood within 100 yards of campground may be used

▓ **Alcohol:** Permitted

▓ **Vehicles:** Up to 30 feet

▓ **Other:** Tent pads required; quiet time 10 p.m.–6 a.m.; maximum 6 people, 2 vehicles per site; firearms prohibited

a short distance west of the campground on US 501. Cyclists, note that bikes may not be ridden on trails alongside the Blue Ridge Parkway; ride only on paved areas.

The James River follows the course of Virginia history, just as it has served as a major west-to-east transportation conduit since the first settlers followed it from the Chesapeake Bay to the site of Jamestown in 1607. The original plan was for the river to extend from Richmond to the Ohio River, but the James and Kanawha Canal only

made it as far west as Buchanan, Virginia. Plan to cross the walkway over the James River and visit the rebuilt Lock No. 7 opposite the Otter Creek Visitor Center. The Battery Creek lock is typical of the 90 locks that were constructed on the canal. This one in particular operated from 1851 to 1880, but the first section of the canal system was built at the falls in Richmond in 1795. Take a short walk on the Trail of Trees, or plan a picnic lunch next to the visitor center along the banks of the James.

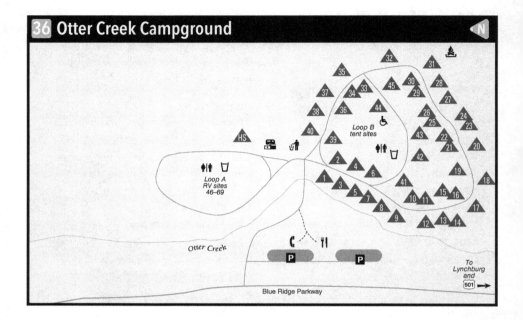

## :: Getting There

From Lynchburg, take US 501 west to the Blue Ridge Parkway at mile 63.8. Enter the parkway and drive north to the Otter Creek Restaurant and adjacent campground at mile 60.9.

**GPS COORDINATES**  N37° 34.620  W79° 20.249

# 37

# Peaks of Otter Campground

*Peaks of Otter offers a tremendous place to camp for those touring the Blue Ridge Parkway.*

**//The mountains** of the Blue Ridge, and of these the Peaks of Otter, are thought to be of a greater height, measured from their base, than any others in our country, and perhaps in North America." So said Thomas Jefferson in his only book, *Notes on the State of Virginia*. Given his expertise in architecture, law, politics, languages, and other fields, we'll have to forgive this bit of overstatement regarding the relative heights of Sharp Top and Flat Top, which stand at 3,875 feet and 4,001 feet, respectively. Given the manner in which they stand apart so geographically from their surroundings, it's easy to see how Charlottesville's favorite son could have embellished their stature a bit.

However, it's difficult to overstate the beauty of the 469-mile Blue Ridge Parkway that stretches from Afton Mountain in Virginia to Cherokee, North Carolina. It's surely one of the most beautiful roads in America, and the Peaks of Otter Campground, located at milepost 86, offers a tremendous place to pitch a tent for those passing through or intent on this as their final destination.

## :: Ratings

BEAUTY: ★ ★ ★
SITE PRIVACY: ★ ★ ★
SPACIOUSNESS: ★ ★ ★ ★
QUIET: ★ ★ ★ ★
SECURITY: ★ ★ ★
CLEANLINESS: ★ ★ ★ ★

Across the road is the picturesque Peaks of Otter Lodge, its reflection mirrored by Abbott Lake. You may want to sample the renowned bounty at the lodge should you tire of camp fare.

The campground's 144 sites are divided among three loops designated as loop A, loop B, and the trailer loop. If you've gotten fed up with campgrounds that offer larger, more private, or more abundant sites for RV users, then you'll love the campground at the Peaks of Otter. There are only 52 sites in the trailer loop, with an additional 4 trailer sites in loop A. The campground features no electric or water hookups, the RV sites are similar in size to the tent sites, and the only concession to vehicle camping is larger parking spots or pull-throughs. How's that for egalitarian camping?

The campground is located in the woods on the flanks of Sharp Top Mountain. While some sites on loop A border VA 43, which crosses the parkway here, the majority lie on the interior of the campground loop. The most private sites are on the upper side of the loop road, notably sites A19, 20, 23, 25, 29, 30, 35–38, and 42. The concession for additional privacy, however, is a 20-foot walk from your car to your tent up the slope of the mountain. The pattern is the same in loop B with sites B1, 3, 4, 7, 8, 10, 13, 16, 20, 21, and 22 providing the most privacy with some additional aerobic exercise thrown in gratis.

## :: Key Information

**ADDRESS:** Blue Ridge Parkway, 10454 Peaks Road, Bedford VA 24523

**OPERATED BY:** National Park Service

**CONTACT:** 540-586-7321; nps.gov/blri

**OPEN:** May 1–Oct. 31; occasional reduced-fee, reduced-service winter camping available

**SITES:** 144

**SITE AMENITIES:** Fire grill, picnic table, lantern pole

**ASSIGNMENT:** Make reservations at recreation.gov; first come, first served

**REGISTRATION:** On site

**FACILITIES:** Water, camp store, flush toilets

**PARKING:** At campsites

**FEE:** $16–$19 per night (varies by season)

**ELEVATION:** 2,600 feet

**RESTRICTIONS:**

▦ **Pets:** Must be attended and on leash shorter than 6 feet; clean up after pet

▦ **Fires:** Use camp stoves and fireplaces; deadwood within 100 yards of campground may be used

▦ **Alcohol:** Permitted

▦ **Vehicles:** Up to 30 feet on pull-through sites

▦ **Other:** Tents must be set up on tent pads; quiet time 10 p.m.–6 a.m.; maximum 6 people, 2 vehicles per site; firearms prohibited

Indigenous people are thought to have passed through Peaks of Otter 8,000 years ago. The first Europeans appeared by the mid-1700s, and an inn opened here in 1834. Many visitors to the region plan their visit during the beginning of June, when the wild rhododendron and mountain laurel are in bloom, but each season has its own characteristic beauty.

A number of area trails graded easy to strenuous begin nearby. The 1-mile loop around Abbott Lake located across VA 43 from the campground falls into the former category, while the 1.5-mile (one-way) hike up to the top of Sharp Top is strenuous. The views from the top are worth the effort, and a bus also makes the trip during summer

months. You'd be remiss, however, if you didn't also take the 4.4-mile (one-way) climb to the top of Flat Top. The Flat Top and Fallingwater Cascades Trails were designated as national recreation trails in 1982 and together offer both spectacular scenery from the series of falls and panoramic views from the top. You can also pick up several trails at the visitor center, located on the other side of the Blue Ridge Parkway from the campground. These include the 0.8-mile Elk Run Trail, the 2.1-mile Johnson Farm Trail, and the 3.3-mile Harkening Hill Trail, all of which are loops. A number of other trails adjoin the Appalachian Trail and are accessible some 5 miles south of the peaks on the Blue Ridge Parkway.

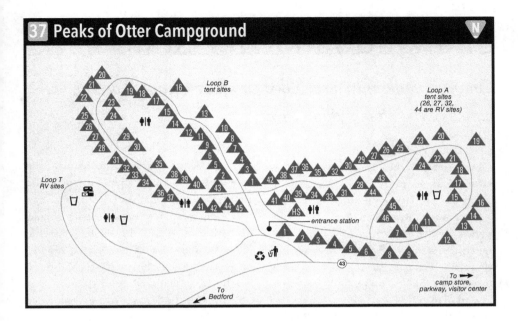

## :: Getting There

Take the Blue Ridge Parkway to its intersection with VA 43 at milepost 86, and go 0.25 mile south on VA 43 to the campground entrance.

**GPS COORDINATES**   N37° 26.613  W79° 36.307

# 38

# Shenandoah River State Park

*Canoe or walk in to a secluded campsite situated on the banks of the Shenandoah River.*

**J**ust down the mountain from the northern entrance to Skyline Drive is the 1,604-acre Raymond R. "Andy" Guest Jr. Shenandoah River State Park. This park, named for the late Virginia local delegate, lies in the shadow of nearby Massanutten Mountain. Planners have learned a thing or two since the first six Virginia parks were created in 1936, and they put this knowledge to use before opening Shenandoah River in 1999. The park's picnic areas, trails, overlooks, boat launch, and campground are all designed to protect the environment. Even the campsite lantern poles have an au naturel look to them. Access to the riverfront is limited. Garbage must be removed by the park visitor. All facilities, including trails, are universally accessible.

Brochures and signs remind campers at River Right Campground to practice minimal-impact camping. The 10 sites are for tent campers only, and there are no drive-in sites; campers must canoe or walk in to their trash-free riverside campsite. All refuse must be taken to the dumpsters at Three Bends Overlook, located near the contact station at the main entrance. The campground has a central parking area with only 21 spaces; extra vehicles should be parked at one of the shelter or picnic lots. The shaded sites are located around an unpaved wood-chip loop trail, and there is a hutch at the parking lot that contains wagons. Use the wagons to transport your gear, and be sure to return them after you've set up camp. A separate hutch houses firewood, where stocked bundles are sold on the honor system. Canoe-in campers should reserve a site ahead of time and note that the campground is located at mile marker 32, 4 miles downstream from a low-water bridge.

Tent pads are palatial compared to similar sites throughout the region, and sites are widely spaced with riparian buffers to provide privacy. Four sites are directly on the riverfront, but the sites set farther back in the forest are scenic and secluded. A bathhouse with running water, showers, and a utility sink sits at the edge of the parking area, making these 10 coveted sites even more desirable. Reservations are a must at this small campground, but individual sites cannot be booked; you must choose from available sites. Canoe or walk in early.

While the 10 wooded sites will be the first choice for most tent campers, Shenandoah River State Park also features a 32-site campground with electric and water hookups at each site. While geared more toward

## :: Ratings

BEAUTY: ★ ★ ★ ★
SITE PRIVACY: ★ ★ ★ ★
SPACIOUSNESS: ★ ★ ★ ★
QUIET: ★ ★ ★ ★
SECURITY: ★ ★ ★ ★
CLEANLINESS: ★ ★ ★ ★ ★

## :: Key Information

**ADDRESS:** Daughter of Stars Drive, P.O. Box 235, Bentonville, VA 22610

**OPERATED BY:** Virginia State Department of Conservation and Recreation

**CONTACT:** 540-622-6840; virginiastateparks.gov

**OPEN:** Year-round, weather permitting

**SITES:** 10 standard; 32 with electric/water hookups

**SITE AMENITIES:** Picnic table, fire grill, lantern pole

**ASSIGNMENT:** First come, first served

**REGISTRATION:** Call 800-933-PARK or visit reserveamerica.com; site assignment on arrival

**FACILITIES:** Boat launch onto Shenandoah River, cabin rental, equestrian trails, fishing, water, hot showers, dish sink, flush and vault toilets, wagons, canoe launch

**PARKING:** Central parking area; equestrian parking

**FEE:** Standard tent site $20 per night; $32 per night with electric/water hookups

**ELEVATION:** 600 feet

**RESTRICTIONS:**
■ **Pets:** On leash; clean up after pet; $5 surcharge

■ **Fires:** Only in camp stoves and fireplaces

■ **Alcohol:** Prohibited

■ **Vehicles:** None at sites, walk-in only

■ **Other:** Use trash bins at Three Bends Overlook; use designated river access points; no cutting live vegetation; quiet hours 10 p.m.–8 a.m.

RV campers, the smaller sites located on the lower loop and designated 19–32 may be just the ticket.

Canoes cannot be rented at the park itself, but plenty of nearby commercial outfitters supply canoes. The National Forest Service runs nine primitive canoe-in campsites along the Shenandoah River for those who want to rough it. Sites are strictly "leave no trace" and are located at mile markers 6, 8–9, 12–14.5, 16–19, and 24–25. Front Royal Canoe (**frontroyalcanoe.com**), Shenandoah River Outfitters (**shenandoahriver.com**), and Downriver Canoe Company (**downriver.com**) are nearby companies that rent canoes, kayaks, and inner tubes as well as arrange shuttles.

Once you're finished canoeing, there are plenty of options available. Shenandoah National Park and Fort Valley are both nearby, as are the towns of Luray and Front Royal. Twenty-four miles of trails crisscross Shenandoah River State Park, 7 miles of which are multiuse. You can hike, bike, or ride along the easy 2.5-mile River Trail, hugging the Shenandoah's South Fork, or you can choose a more challenging hike through the forest. A private company offers horseback interpretive trail rides from their stable; watch for signs as you descend the windy drive from the entrance contact station. There is a designated equestrian parking lot, and certain trails are designated for horses.

The park also offers a number of options with real roofs and indoor plumbing, including a six-bedroom lodge, two- and three-bedroom cabins, and camp cabins. These are also available by reservation at **reserveamerica.com.**

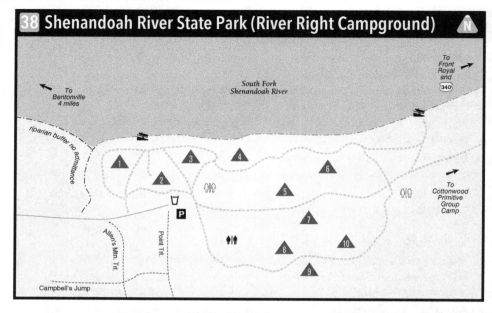

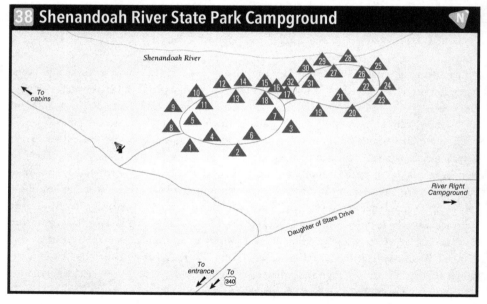

## :: Getting There

From I-66, take Exit 6 to Front Royal. Turn right onto US 340. The park is located 8 miles south on US 340.

**GPS COORDINATES**  N38° 51.764  W78° 18.177

# 39

# Sherando Lake Recreation Area

*Sherando is thought to be a variant on "Shenandoah."*

**While living** in the Shenandoah Valley for 20 years, I took Sherando Lake Recreation Area largely for granted. It was just a half-hour's drive from my home, and I enjoyed visiting for a day of swimming, fishing, canoeing, or mountain biking but infrequently spent the night. In the course of compiling information for this book, however, I saw Sherando Lake in a new light when I compared it to other beautiful campgrounds across Virginia. The name, Sherando, is thought to be a variant on "Shenandoah," which is widely translated as "daughter of the stars." And the campground here shines brightly as a possible destination for campers, not only because of its own offerings but also because of its potential as a base camp from which to explore this section of the George Washington and Jefferson National Forests, the Blue Ridge Parkway, and the Shenandoah Valley.

Nothing, to my mind, is as beautiful as a lake set against a mountainous background. Sherando Lake Recreation Area is tucked up against the side of the Blue Ridge Mountains on the eastern edge of the Shenandoah Valley. Turning off VA 664, you'll drive 2.5 miles on the hard-surface road that passes the beach and day-use area before passing campgrounds A, B, and C and finally ending at the group campground. Of the first three, campground A (White Oak Campground) is the most inviting and is limited to tents, pop-ups, and trailers that are less than 25 feet long. Situated on a hillside of dense oak trees, the 34 sites along this loop are spacious and shady, offering more than enough privacy between you and your neighbors. The sites have been renovated, but you'll still find some of the original stonework from the park's construction by CCC workers in the 1930s. To really admire their accomplishments at Sherando, take a close look at the stone beachfront bathhouse and pavilion.

The River Bend Campground, aka campground B, lies along the South River (actually a creek), which runs through this recreation area. It is flat, open, and the only loop that has hookups for RVs. A little farther down the road is the Meadow Loop, or campground C, with 18 sites that are flat and open and lack hookups. Campsites in loop C and the lower portion of loop A are reservable at **www.fs.usda.gov/gwj.**

There are actually two lakes at Sherando. The 7-acre Upper Sherando Lake, near the end of the main park road, was created by the Soil Conservation Service in the 1960s and is designated for fishing. Both

## :: Ratings

BEAUTY: ★ ★ ★ ★ ★
SITE PRIVACY: ★ ★ ★ ★ ★
SPACIOUSNESS: ★ ★ ★ ★ ★
QUIET: ★ ★ ★ ★
SECURITY: ★ ★ ★ ★ ★
CLEANLINESS: ★ ★ ★ ★

## :: Key Information

**ADDRESS:** Glenwood-Pedlar Ranger District, P.O. Box 10, Natural Bridge Station, VA 24579

**OPERATED BY:** U.S. Forest Service

**CONTACT:** 540-291-2188; www.fs.usda.gov/gwj

**OPEN:** April 1–end of October

**SITES:** 65

**SITE AMENITIES:** Picnic table, fire grill, lantern pole

**ASSIGNMENT:** Reserve at recreation .gov; on-site selection

**REGISTRATION:** On arrival

**FACILITIES:** Lake swimming, boating, and fishing; water; flush toilets; hot showers in campground and in lake bathhouse; drink machines

**PARKING:** At campsites, picnic area, and lake

**FEE:** $20 per night; $25 per night with hookups

**ELEVATION:** 1,860 feet

**RESTRICTIONS:**
▪ **Pets:** On leash and attended at all times; not allowed on beach or in swimming areas

▪ **Fires:** Only in camp stoves and grills; must be attended

▪ **Alcohol:** Permitted at campsite only

▪ **Vehicles:** Must remain in designated campsite area

▪ **Other:** Quiet hours 10 p.m.–6 a.m.; maximum stay is 21 consecutive days; swimming and picnic areas close at dark

lakes are stocked with trout in the spring and fall by the Virginia Department of Game and Inland Fisheries. All of the appropriate licenses are required to fish year-round. The 25-acre lower lake has an attractive swimming beach with a roped-off wading area. Stronger swimmers can practice their strokes on the way out to an island that is approximately a quarter mile from the beach. Anglers can cast a line anywhere along the shore away from the beach, although many choose to do so at the lower end of the lake by the dam. The Lakeside Trail will take you there, as will a turnoff from the camp road 1 mile after the entrance station.

Hikers and mountain bikers will find much to do at Sherando Lake, as they explore trails that meander, as well as those that climb up the surrounding mountains to the famed Blue Ridge Parkway. After passing site 5 on campground A loop, you'll notice the well-blazed Blue Loop Trail, which goes 0.5 mile to Lookout Rock and connects with other trails for longer and more strenuous climbs, including a 4-mile ascent (one-way) to Bald Mountain. The White Rock Gap Trail is a favorite among mountain bikers as a way to ascend and descend to and from the Blue Ridge Parkway. Whether you're looking for a little quiet time in the woods or a place to let the kids swim while you explore outdoor recreational pursuits, you're sure to find something enjoyable at Sherando Lake.

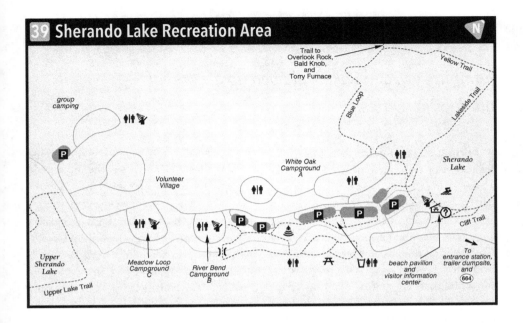

## :: Getting There

From I-64, take the exit for Sherando Lake, located at the bottom of the western slope of Afton Mountain. Drive 2 miles on VA 624, and then veer right at the bend onto VA 664. Continue 8 miles to the recreation entrance on the right.

**GPS COORDINATES**   N37° 55.179  W79° 00.485

# 40

# Todd Lake Recreation Area

*Camping at Todd Lake will open up a world of outdoor activities.*

**L**iving just a half-hour's drive from Todd Lake over the course of my 20 years as a Shenandoah Valley resident, I confess to having spent more time at this recreation area taking a dip in the 7.5-acre lake after a rigorous mountain bike ride or a daylong family outing than as an overnight camper. No matter how far away you live, however, you'll find that camping at Todd Lake opens up a world of outdoor activities in this part of the George Washington and Jefferson National Forests. Forest Service representatives suggest that campers looking for optimal seclusion at this or any other national forest campground should plan their visit during midweek or outside of the busy summer months.

This recreation area is located southwest of Harrisonburg. After a short ride through some of the Shenandoah Valley's most endearing back roads, you'll enter the Todd Lake Recreation Area from FDR 95, where the road turns from hard surface to gravel. The campground sits on a knoll to the left of the main road, with the day-use area straight ahead just inside the gated entrance. After a short downhill, you'll see the large parking area for the lake on the right. Continue past here for access to the expansive wooded picnic area that ends at the edge of the lake. There's a roped-off sand beach and swimming area, and the additional lake area is available for anglers and nonmotorized boats. Boaters and anglers looking for a little more elbow room will drive a few miles to the larger Elkhorn Lake.

Half of Todd Lake's 20 campsites (1–4, 16–20) are spaced along the straight part of the camp road, and the other half (5–15) along a loop at the end. The sites are as spacious as any that I've seen at campgrounds in the Old Dominion, and the feeling is enhanced by the dense second-growth oak and white pines that permeate the area. Sites 12–20 are also surrounded by stands of mountain laurel. If that's not enough privacy, however, plan to visit during the week, and head for site 12, which lies at the end of the campground loop with additional seclusion provided by high dirt berms. There are no bad sites at this campground.

A short walk down the foot trail located between sites 3 and 4 leads to the picnic area, beach, and lake. Plan to enjoy a meal alfresco in the heavily wooded picnic area by the lake, even though you have cooking facilities back at the campsite.

Hiking opportunities abound in the Todd Lake Area as in the rest of the George

## :: Ratings

BEAUTY: ★ ★ ★ ★
SITE PRIVACY: ★ ★ ★
SPACIOUSNESS: ★ ★ ★ ★ ★
QUIET: ★ ★ ★
SECURITY: ★ ★ ★
CLEANLINESS: ★ ★ ★ ★

# :: Key Information

**ADDRESS:** North River Ranger District, 401 Oakwood Drive, Harrisonburg, VA 22801

**OPERATED BY:** U.S. Forest Service

**CONTACT:** 540-432-0187; www.fs.usda.gov/gwj

**OPEN:** Mid-May–mid-November

**SITES:** 20

**SITE AMENITIES:** Fire ring, picnic table, lantern post

**ASSIGNMENT:** First come, first served; no reservations

**REGISTRATION:** Self-registration on site

**FACILITIES:** Hot showers, flush toilets, lake swimming, potable water

**PARKING:** At campsite and day-use area at lake

**FEE:** $16 per night (includes beach and picnic fees)

**ELEVATION:** 2,000 feet

**RESTRICTIONS:**
■ **Pets:** On leash, attended, and under control at all times; not allowed at beach

■ **Fires:** Use fire rings, stoves, grills, and fireplaces

■ **Alcohol:** No restriction at campground; not allowed at beach

■ **Vehicles:** Up to 21 feet

■ **Other:** Campsite must be occupied the first night; must be attended within a 24-hour period; 21-day maximum length of stay

Washington and Jefferson National Forests. A 1-mile leg stretcher loops Todd Lake, while the 4-mile Trimble Mountain Trail can be found on the opposite side of FDR 95 near the dump station. This loop follows the side of the mountain but should not be too challenging for those of average fitness.

If you're looking for a real workout, drive on the hard-surface section of FDR 95 to reach the trailhead of the 25.6-mile Wild Oak National Recreation Trail. Don't let the distance or the terrain discourage you. Besides the trailhead, this trail intersects with forest roads in two other places, offering three point-to-point day hikes. Segment A is 10.2 miles and climbs to the trail's highest point at 4,351 feet atop Little Bald Knob before descending to the North

River (a creek, really) and the former site of a stockman's camp known as Camp Todd. Section B's 5.2 miles are said to be the most strenuous, as the trail climbs slopes of up to 46% for a total of more than 1,700 feet before reaching FDR 96. Section C is 10.2 miles and traverses Hankey Mountain's relatively gentle slopes before crossing a steeper and rockier Lookout Mountain.

Area mountain biking opportunities are unlimited if you combine existing trails and Forest Service roads. I've long enjoyed the 14-mile Great Lakes Loop that passes Todd Lake on gravel roads. Start from Todd Lake, heading uphill on FDR 95A before circling back on FDR 95 along a series of challenging ascents and exhilarating descents that take you past Elkhorn Lake and the Staunton Dam.

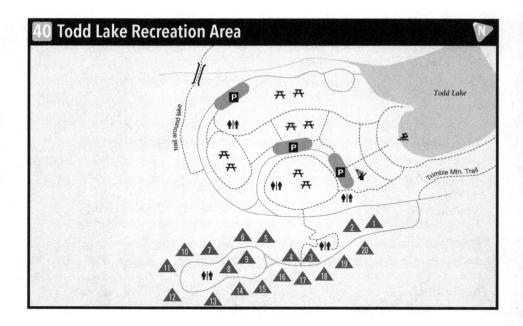

## :: Getting There

From Bridgewater, follow VA 42 for 3 miles south to Mossy Creek. Continue on VA 747 where VA 42 bends sharply to the left. Take VA 731 for 1 mile before turning left onto VA 730. Go 3 miles and turn right onto VA 718. Follow this for a mile until it turns into FDR 95. Continue on FDR 95 for 2 miles to the entrance to Todd Lake.

**GPS COORDINATES** N38° 21.870 W79° 12.534

# Southwest Virginia

# 41

# Breaks Interstate Park

*Breaks Interstate Park on the Virginia–Kentucky border features one of the largest canyons east of the Mississippi.*

**B**reaks Interstate Park is so far southwest that it is almost east—in eastern Kentucky, that is. Put another way, this park sits closer to the state capitals of Kentucky, Tennessee, and North Carolina than to Virginia's capital in Richmond. This 4,500-acre park, which features the largest canyon east of the Mississippi, sits on the Virginia–Kentucky border almost as far west as Detroit. Rather than having one state manage the shared park, the two teamed up and formed a partnership. The Breaks Interstate Commission administers the parkland via a concessionaire. The good news is that if you've come a distance to stay at Breaks Interstate Park, you'll be glad you did. Whether it's working up a sweat on the hiking/biking trails, beating the heat at Splash! in the Park, whitewater rafting through the Breaks Gorge on the Russel Fork River, chasing a little white ball at nearby Willowbrook Country Club, or sitting back and enjoying musical shows at the park's amphitheater, there truly is something for everybody here.

## :: Ratings

BEAUTY: ★ ★ ★
SITE PRIVACY: ★ ★ ★
SPACIOUSNESS: ★ ★ ★
QUIET: ★ ★
SECURITY: ★ ★ ★ ★
CLEANLINESS: ★ ★ ★

There are 138 campsites in seven spurs and loops. An eighth spur is dedicated to tents or groups, unless the campground is full, at which point the access road is unblocked and the spur is designated "overflow camping." There are a lot of sites and the park can get crowded, but the rambling campground has no shortage of space. Besides the 16 overflow shaded tent sites, 15 sites are dedicated to tent camping.

The remaining sites have either electrical access, or water and electric hookups. The spur encompassing sites 66–80 has full hookups, including sewer, so tent campers should avoid this area. Twenty other sites offer complete hookups as well, but most of them are integrated into the campground and clearly marked. The campground features other conveniences too, including laundry rooms, vending machines, and a camp store. These amenities are suitably rustic, although Breaks is more commercial than most public parks, with a 70-room lodge, a conference center, four vacation cottages, and a gift shop.

Breaks bills itself as "the Grand Canyon of the South." That's a stretch, as the quarter-mile-deep gorge is covered in so much forest that the drama of the scene is tempered. It appears to be a panoramic wooded valley rather than a canyon chiseled out by erosion. Regardless, it offers stunning views along with a variety of outdoor adventures.

## :: Key Information

**ADDRESS:** 627 Commission Circle, Breaks, VA 24607

**OPERATED BY:** Breaks Interstate Commission

**CONTACT:** 276-865-4413; breakspark.com

**OPEN:** March–first Monday in December

**SITES:** 138

**SITE AMENITIES:** Picnic table, fire grill

**ASSIGNMENT:** First come, first served

**REGISTRATION:** Call 800-933-PARK or visit reserveamerica.com; site assignment on arrival

**FACILITIES:** Cabin rental, water park, whitewater rafting, fishing, boating, playground, amphitheater, camp store, laundry, vending machines, restaurant, flush toilets, showers

**PARKING:** 2 vehicles in addition to camping unit at site

**FEE:** standard tent site $15 per night; $22 per night with electric/water hookups; $24 per night with electricity, water, and sewer

**ELEVATION:** 1,600 feet

**RESTRICTIONS:**

■ **Pets:** Must be on leash

■ **Fires:** Only in designated areas; firewood can be purchased at park but should not be brought in so as not to introduce wood-boring insects

■ **Alcohol:** Prohibited

■ **Vehicles:** Up to 40 feet

■ **Other:** Maximum 6 people, 2 vehicles per site; maximum stay is 14 consecutive nights; quiet hours 10 p.m.–6 a.m.

There are 25 miles of trails in the park, mainly consisting of short ones that can be combined to form longer treks. The Mountain Bike Trail loops can be combined to create 12 miles of moderate to difficult riding through some outstanding scenery. The park convenience store rents bikes, which can also be used on park roads. Grassy Overlook Trail can be accessed from between sites 10 and 11 in section B of the campground. Overlook Trail, which hugs the edge of cliffs, is popular in spring and fall. Other activities include horseback riding and pool swimming, along with boating and fishing on the central 12-acre Laurel Lake or on the trout-stocked Russell Fork River. Additionally, whitewater rafting is popular in October, when water released from Flanagan Reservoir creates Class IV–Class VI rapids.

Also popular, especially with nonhikers, is the nearby Cumberland Mountain View Drive. It is a 19-mile panoramic trip along VA 611, between Breaks Interstate Park and Clintwood, Virginia. Parts of the road are unpaved, and there are several sharp turns, so allow several hours for the trip.

Daniel Boone is credited with discovering Breaks. He is mentioned in the small museum located at the visitor center. Exhibits also detail the unique geology that caused the sandstone erosion, as well as the formation of coal and process of coal mining—past and present—in the local hills. Just outside the visitor center are a working mill and a nonworking moonshine still. The region is full of stories about mountain folk, including the infamous Hatfield–McCoy feud, which is said to have occurred nearby.

Wildflowers are a key attraction at Breaks, where blooming dogwoods dazzle hikers in spring and rhododendron blossoms in early summer. Autumn leaves

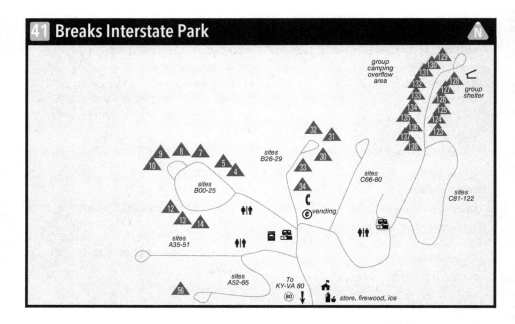

bring spectators as well, as the dramatic reds and yellows enhance views from scenic overlooks. The Towers is the most famous of the overlooks, and while viewing the plunging canyons cut out by the river over years of erosion, one can see why Daniel Boone turned back in 1767. Fortunately, access to Breaks Interstate Park is easier today.

While it may seem like blasphemy to inveterate tent campers, I have learned that age (and a bad back) is oft accompanied by an appreciation for indoor plumbing, a proper bed, and hard roof, underneath which rain can actually be enjoyed. Be sure to check out this park's array of camping cabins, two- and three-bedroom cabins, and multibedroom lodges.

## :: Getting There

From Wytheville, take I-77 North to East River Mountain Tunnel. Go through the tunnel and then west on US 460. At Vansant, turn left onto VA 83. At Haysi, turn right onto KY-VA 80. The park entrance is 8 miles ahead on the left.

**GPS COORDINATES**   N37° 17.592  W82° 17.819

# 42

# Cave Springs Recreation Area

*The quarter-acre, spring-fed pond at Cave Springs is a great destination.*

**Far out** in the southwest corner of Virginia is an area known for coal production but largely overlooked by the rest of the state. Its topography of horizontal Appalachian Plateau sandstone identifies it less with Virginia and more with neighboring Kentucky, Tennessee, and West Virginia. Local residents are known for their tenacity in carving out lives from largely inhospitable landscapes. Early timber and mining efforts stripped many of these mountains, and the Forest Service bought land for the Clinch Ranger District to protect the headwaters of the Tennessee River. Visit this little-known region, and you'll be amazed by the natural beauty that lies in this obscure corner of the Old Dominion.

Cave Springs Recreation Area is one of those scarcely visited gems harbored in Virginia's national forests. It lies at the foot of Stone Mountain, which is part of Cumberland Mountain, forming the border with Kentucky. Most people don't even know that Virginia shares a border with the Bluegrass State. While few Virginians make the drive out to the Clinch Ranger District, those lucky enough to live nearby or in the neighboring states of Kentucky and Tennessee can savor this outstanding camping destination.

After passing through a rolling agricultural landscape, you'll find this wooded oasis where dense stands of holly hug the quarter-acre, spring-fed pond. Cave Springs is particularly appealing during the heat of the summer. The entire recreation area is shaded by a canopy of hemlocks, and the spring-fed pond stays below 72°F. Those looking to take a cool dip—a very cool dip—need look no further. The campground's 41 sites are private and well spaced along a single loop. All sites provide the private getaways that you'd expect from this campground. The narrow campground roads help minimize RV use as well. Native stone walls constructed by Forest Service employees and senior citizens in the 1960s snake through the area, along with wild rhododendron.

The 1-mile Cave Overlook Trail loop will take you to the cave from which the area and springs derive their name. Spelunkers may be disappointed that the cave is not open to the public, but it's still a nice walk. Hikers looking for a strenuous outing can begin the 14.3-mile (point-to-point) Stone Mountain Trail at the Cave Springs Recreation Area. The cascading waters of Roaring

## :: Ratings

BEAUTY: ★ ★ ★ ★
SITE PRIVACY: ★ ★ ★ ★
SPACIOUSNESS: ★ ★ ★ ★ ★
QUIET: ★ ★ ★
SECURITY: ★ ★ ★
CLEANLINESS: ★ ★ ★

## :: Key Information

**ADDRESS:** Clinch Ranger District, 9416 Darden Drive, Wise, VA 24293

**OPERATED BY:** U.S. Forest Service

**CONTACT:** 276-328-2931; www.fs.usda.gov/gwj

**OPEN:** May 15–Sept.15

**SITES:** 41

**SITE AMENITIES:** Picnic table, fire grill, lantern pole

**ASSIGNMENT:** First come, first served

**REGISTRATION:** On arrival

**FACILITIES:** Water, warm showers, flush toilets

**PARKING:** At campsite and small day-use area

**FEE:** $12 per night

**ELEVATION:** 1,380 feet

**RESTRICTIONS:**
■ **Pets:** On leash and attended
■ **Fires:** In camp stoves and fireplaces only; dead and down wood may be collected; no cutting or damaging live or standing dead trees
■ **Alcohol:** Prohibited
■ **Vehicles:** 22 feet
■ **Other:** Campsites should not be left unattended for a 24-hour period; quiet hours 10 p.m.–6 a.m.

Run and outstanding views of Virginia and Kentucky peaks make this trek well worth the effort. Along the way, you'll pass through old-growth hemlock that is more than 300 years old. A 1-mile side trip from Olinger Gap will take you to Lake Keokee for some fishing or additional sightseeing.

The 92-acre Lake Keokee offers fishing for tiger muskie, largemouth bass, catfish, and sunfish, as well as limited picnicking facilities. Bring a canoe to enjoy a quiet paddle around a lake with a number of interesting coves—gasoline motors are prohibited.

Another option is to circle the lake on the fairly tame 3-mile Lake Keokee Loop Trail.

Cave Springs Recreation Area lies farther from most Virginians than other destinations in these pages. But don't let that stop you from putting aside the popular misconceptions regarding this region's socioeconomic status. This beautiful land features cool, quiet campgrounds when the rest of the state is blasted by heat. Camp at Cave Springs, bask in the cool waters, hike the mountains, and discover all that's so refreshing about a part of Virginia that many Virginians have forgotten.

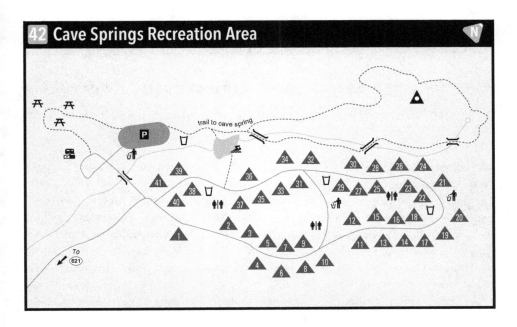

## :: Getting There

From Big Stone Gap, follow US Alt. 58 west 3 miles to VA 621. Turn right onto VA 621, and follow it 6.5 miles to the sign for Cave Springs.

**GPS COORDINATES**   N36° 47.998  W82° 55.450

# Claytor Lake State Park

*As one of Virginia's state parks with a marina, Claytor Lake is a natural destination for boaters and anglers.*

**C**laytor Lake State Park lies on the 4,500-acre, 21-mile-long Claytor Lake. The lake was formed in 1939 with the damming of the New River, just south of Radford, by the Appalachian Power Company. The New River flows in a northerly direction and is thought to be the second-oldest river in the world. The park came under the operation of Virginia's Division of State Parks in 1951. As one of Virginia's state parks with a marina, Claytor Lake State Park is a natural destination for boaters and anglers. The park offers bicycle and boat rentals, as well as a selection of supplies for water sports. Motorboating and fishing on the lake are this park's greatest draws. Bass, catfish, muskie, and walleye are the favorite catches of anglers. In addition, the 450-foot sandy beach and five group picnic shelters provide activities for landlubbers. Those without boats will find a number of excellent coves along the shoreline from which to fish. However, the four campground loops offer the option of sleeping out under the trees, whether or not you've towed your boat and brought your rod and reel.

After passing the contact station, you'll see the campground entrance on the right. Signs will direct you to loops A and B on the right and loops C and D on the left. The sites in loops A, B, and C are large, with a fine gravel surface bounded by landscape timbers, but they offer no electric hookups. Tent campers should be sure to bring a ground cloth and mattress pad. The canopy of mature pines and hardwoods creates considerable shade for loops A, B, and C, although there is minimal understory for privacy between sites. For more privacy, have a look at sites A9–27, which are flat but laid out on a hillside.

Loop D has a different feel than A, B, or C. In addition to being positioned along a flat, open area, it's the only one without delineated tent pads. Loop D sites are laid out along three lines, but D30–34 are the most secluded, with the dirt access road in front and a buffer of pine trees behind. Despite its appearance as more conducive to tent camping than the other loops, it's also the only one with electric hookups and is geared toward RVs. Go figure.

The park has seven picnic shelters and one gazebo that are available for rent, and 4 miles of trails for easy walks and bicycle rides through the woods. You can pick up the 1.6-mile Claytor Lake Trail across from site C4, while the 0.6-mile Shady Ridge Trail

## :: Ratings

BEAUTY: ★ ★ ★
SITE PRIVACY: ★ ★ ★
SPACIOUSNESS: ★ ★ ★
QUIET: ★ ★ ★
SECURITY: ★ ★ ★
CLEANLINESS: ★ ★ ★

## :: Key Information

**ADDRESS:** 6620 Ben H. Bolen Drive, Dublin, VA 24084

**OPERATED BY:** Virginia Department of Conservation and Recreation

**CONTACT:** 540-643-2500; virginiastateparks.gov

**OPEN:** April 1–Dec. 1

**SITES:** 110

**SITE AMENITIES:** Picnic table, fire grill, lantern pole

**ASSIGNMENT:** First come, first served

**REGISTRATION:** Call 800-933-PARK or visit reserveamerica.com; site assignment on arrival

**FACILITIES:** Cabin and lodge rental; full-service marina; lake boating, fishing, and swimming; flush toilets; hot showers; pay phone; drink machines at marina

**PARKING:** 2 vehicles in addition to camping unit; extra parking available

**FEE:** Standard tent site $20 per night; $27 per night with electric/water hookups

**ELEVATION:** 1,900 feet

**RESTRICTIONS:**

■ **Pets:** Must be on short leash or enclosed

■ **Fires:** Only in camp stoves and fire rings

■ **Alcohol:** Public use is prohibited

■ **Vehicles:** Up to 35 feet

■ **Other:** Swimming only in designated areas Memorial Day–Labor Day; no cutting trees; no washing dishes in restroom sinks

---

is accessible from the picnic area. Mountain bikers may want to use Claytor Lake State Park to ride on the 57-mile New River Trail, part of which runs parallel to the New River near Claytor Lake.

Be sure to stop by the historic Howe House, built between 1876 and 1879 by Haven B. Howe. Besides being a Civil War veteran, Virginia legislator, and talented woodworker, Howe was an early environmentalist who worked to end pollution of the New River by iron ore smelting plants. He was also a proponent of conservation-oriented farming. Howe House was built with brick that had been kiln-dried on the property along with timber felled from the surrounding woods. It now houses the park's visitor center and administrative offices. It contains hands-on exhibits that focus on lake ecology and fish life, as well as the park's Discovery Center, which offers summer environmental education programs. Check at the visitor center to see which guided interpretive programs are going on during your stay at the park.

Over the past couple of years, Virginia's state park system has been busy adding lodgings to parks that did not have them. While it may seem like blasphemy to inveterate tent campers, I have personally learned that age (and a bad back) is oft accompanied by an appreciation for indoor plumbing, a proper bed, and a hard roof, underneath which rain can actually be enjoyed. Be sure to check out this park's array of two- and three-bedroom cabins and multibedroom lodges.

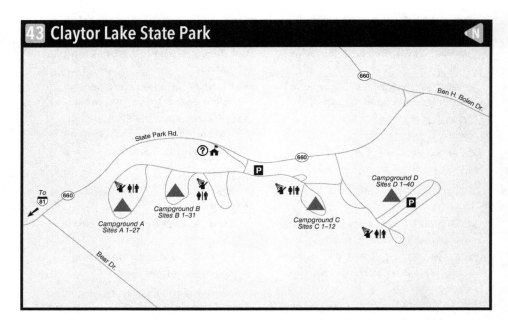

## :: Getting There

From I-81, take Exit 101 and drive 2 miles on VA 660 to the park's entrance.
**GPS COORDINATES**   N37° 03.631  W80° 37.471

# 44

# Comers Rock Campground

*Comers Rock is a suitable alternative for those seeking to be far from the madding crowd.*

**W**ith so many campgrounds in the Mount Rogers National Recreation Area, some might wonder why the low-budget Comers Rock Campground is included here. Its six sites, vault toilet, and location away from the epicenter of outdoor activities in this 119,000-acre national forest recreation area will probably not draw many campers from the larger and spiffier campgrounds, such as Beartree and Grindstone. But these qualities make it a suitable camping alternative for those seeking to be far from the madding crowd and RV campers.

Located a short distance from US 21 on the eastern end of the Mount Rogers NRA, this campground sits along gravel FDR 57. The views from this road running along the ridgeline of Iron Mountain are nothing short of spectacular. Iron Mountain forms a recreational as well as a geologic spine for the area, with this campground situated in a saddle with northern views across the adjacent 2,858-acre Little Dry Run Wilderness. The campsites are haphazardly arranged along a single loop with little vegetation

between them, and some sites are not clearly marked. But they are all separated from each other with varied elevations that provide a modicum of privacy.

A trail next to the single vault toilet connects with the Virginia Highlands Horse Trail, which meanders throughout Mount Rogers NRA along Iron Mountain. This section of the trail is designated multiuse, so hikers and mountain bikers can use the orange-blazed path to take off from their campsites for some outdoor exploration. Given that bikes are not, however, allowed in designated wilderness areas, it's best to begin pedaling west on the trail toward the 5-acre Hale Lake, just 2 miles down the road. Those whose inclinations steer them away from singletrack riding can start pedaling down FDR 57, which ends a short distance down the road, just past the lake at the intersection with VA 672.

As the free forest map for Mount Rogers NRA once stated, "whoever invented mountain bicycles surely had the Mount Rogers National Recreation Area in mind!" There is no shortage of places to ride in these parts. In my book *Mountain Bike! Virginia*, I referred to one of the rides close to Comers Rock Campground as "Mountain Bike Heaven." It's an 8-mile loop that's accessible from FDR 14 on the east side of US 21. You'll earn your aerobic stripes on the 2.6-mile climb, but the 3-mile descent will have you clamoring for another go-round. Between the 33-mile

## :: Ratings

BEAUTY: ★ ★ ★
SITE PRIVACY: ★ ★
SPACIOUSNESS: ★ ★ ★
QUIET: ★ ★ ★
SECURITY: ★ ★
CLEANLINESS: ★ ★ ★

## :: Key Information

**ADDRESS:** Mount Rogers National Recreation Area, 3714 VA 16, Marion, VA 24354

**OPERATED BY:** U.S. Forest Service

**CONTACT:** 276-783-5196; www.fs.usda.gov/gwj

**OPEN:** April 1–Oct. 31

**SITES:** 6

**SITE AMENITIES:** Picnic table, grill, lantern pole

**ASSIGNMENT:** First come, first served

**REGISTRATION:** On site

**FACILITIES:** Water, vault toilet

**PARKING:** At campsite and picnic area

**FEE:** $5 per night

**ELEVATION:** 3,800 feet

**RESTRICTIONS:**
- **Pets:** Must be on leash and attended
- **Fires:** Use available grills
- **Alcohol:** Prohibited
- **Vehicles:** Up to 22 feet
- **Other:** Maximum stay is 21 days in a 30-day period; no cutting live trees; Forest Service does not plow snow

Virginia Creeper Trail and the vast network of forest roads and trails, opportunities for mountain biking here abound. Given its minimal amenities, you're more likely to use your site at Comers Rock Campground as a base from which to explore this 119,000-acre section of the George Washington and Jefferson National Forests.

Mountain bikers are not the only ones who will appreciate the Mount Rogers area. Equestrians will enjoy saddling up and taking in the sights along the Virginia Highlands Horse Trail, which stretches 67 miles (point-to-point) from VA 94 near Ivanhoe to VA 600 at Elk Garden Gap. Trailer parking is available at the Hussy Mountain Horse Camp on FDR 14 along the previously mentioned Mountain Bike Heaven loop, through which the Highlands Horse Trail runs.

Hikers will also find ample places to get close to nature on more than 400 miles of trails that meander through this southwestern corner of the Old Dominion, including 60 miles of Appalachian Trail. The AT goes right through the town of Damascus. Whatever your outdoor interests, you're sure to find places to enjoy it at Mount Rogers.

Mount Rogers NRA has no shortage of superb camping destinations. In addition to those detailed in this book, there are also Beartree Recreation Area (90 sites), Grindstone Recreation Area (108 sites), Raccoon Branch Campground (20 sites), Stony Fork Campground (54 sites), and Fox Creek Horse Campground (32 sites). You can get additional information at **www.fs.usda .gov/gwj**. Once you arrive, be sure to stop by the Mount Rogers ranger station on VA 16 for a district map and trail brochures. When a national forest district has the word "recreation" in its name, you can be sure that camping accommodations and outdoor activities will be awesome.

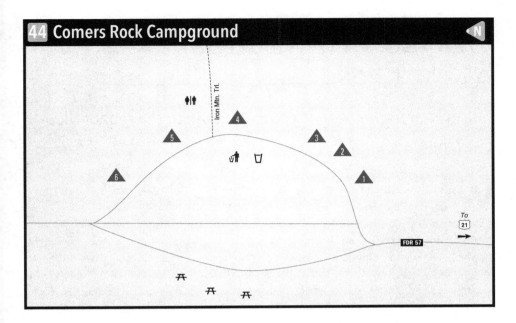

## :: Getting There

From Wytheville, take US 21 through Speedwell, and turn right onto FDR 57 at the top of Iron Mountain. Go 4 miles to the campground.

**GPS COORDINATES**   N36° 45.774  W81° 13.427

# 45

# Grayson Highlands State Park

*The overall feeling is that you're clinging to the roof of the Old Dominion.*

**W**ith **elevations** up to 5,089 feet, Grayson Highlands is the loftiest state park in Virginia. From the highest point at the Pinnacles, you'll find breathtaking views of surrounding mountains, including Mount Rogers (5,729 feet), the tallest peak in Virginia. The overall feeling is not that you're on an isolated elevation but more like you're clinging to the roof of the Old Dominion. Originally known as Mount Rogers State Park, Grayson Highlands became part of the state system in 1965. As you enter the park from US 58 at 3,698 feet and ascend to the visitor center at 4,953 feet, you get the feeling that you're climbing into heaven.

The park office is on the left after the contact station. The campground turnoff is another 2.5 miles by the overnight parking area for backpackers. Grayson Highlands has the distinction of being one of two Virginia State Parks through which the 2,172-mile Appalachian Trail passes on its way between Maine and Georgia. It's a popular spot with thru-hikers, as well as those looking to accumulate some AT mileage.

The campground is isolated, its sites clustered around a grassy, bald knoll. The 73 sites are positioned along two interlocking loops, with considerable differences in privacy and exposure. Past the first bathhouse, the woods become more invasive. At elevations such as this, however, trees have a tough time getting much height. Given a choice, it's definitely worth a drive around to pick out a good site, especially if spending a few days here. Sites 49–59 at the rear of the loop under the shade of overhanging hardwoods are particularly appealing. All sites have gravel bases, so pack a ground cloth and sleeping pad.

Grayson Highland's location on the southern edge of the Mount Rogers National Recreation Area and the Little Wilson Creek Wilderness Area helps attract a considerable number of visitors every year to this 4,822-acre palace among the clouds. Outdoor enthusiasts enjoy various activities, including equestrian facilities, hiking, and mountain bike trails. Backcountry fly-fishermen might enjoy casting a line onto Cabin and Wilson Creeks. These are special regulation areas, so contact park officials for specific rules and license requirements. You might also want to pick up a copy of the park's Mountain Bike Trail Guide or Horse Trail Guide.

## :: Ratings

BEAUTY: ★ ★ ★ ★
SITE PRIVACY: ★ ★ ★
SPACIOUSNESS: ★ ★ ★
QUIET: ★ ★ ★
SECURITY: ★ ★ ★
CLEANLINESS: ★ ★ ★ ★

# :: Key Information

**ADDRESS:** 829 Grayson Highland Lane, Mouth of Wilson, VA 24363

**OPERATED BY:** Virginia Department of Conservation and Recreation

**CONTACT:** 276-579-7092; virginiastateparks.gov

**OPEN:** March–early December

**SITES:** 73

**SITE AMENITIES:** Picnic table, fire ring, lantern pole

**ASSIGNMENT:** First come, first served

**REGISTRATION:** Call 800-933-PARK or visit reserveamerica.com; site assignment on arrival

**FACILITIES:** Equestrian campground

and trails, camping lodge, laundry, camp store, pay phone, hot showers

**PARKING:** At campsite

**FEE:** Standard tent site $20 per night; $27 per night with electric/water hookups

**ELEVATION:** 4,000 feet

**RESTRICTIONS:**

▪ **Pets:** Not allowed in public facilities

▪ **Fires:** In grills, stoves, and fire rings

▪ **Alcohol:** Public use is prohibited

▪ **Vehicles:** No restriction on RV length

▪ **Other:** Maximum stay is 14 consecutive nights in a 30-day period

The visitor center is located near the trailheads for Twin Pinnacles and Listening Rock Trails by the summit of Haw Orchard Mountain. Inside are exhibits of the area's once-volcanic geology and the history of the rough life led by European settlers, including one on the how-tos of whiskey making. The Mountain Crafts Shop, located in this stone and timber building, sells gifts made by local artisans of the Rooftop of Virginia Community Action Program.

Be sure to take the half-hour walk up the Big Pinnacle Trail, which offers incredible views of Virginia's two tallest mountains, Mount Rogers and White Top (5,520 feet), in addition to the surrounding "lowlands" of Virginia, North Carolina, and Tennessee. There are other trails in the park that can be strung together for longer and more varied hikes. Mount Rogers can be reached by taking the Rhododendron Trail from the Massie Gap parking area to the Appalachian Trail and continuing on the AT for a 4-mile

(one-way) hike. The hike is moderately challenging, but don't expect tremendous views from this lofty point. Mount Rogers is capped by spruce trees and offers no views at all.

Many festivals take place at Grayson Highlands March–October. Bluegrass lovers should visit the third Saturday in June, when the Wayne Henderson Music Festival takes place at Grayson Highlands. The park gets crowded, so plan your trip accordingly. Also, keep in mind that the weather can change rapidly here, so pack for extremes of temperature. One balmy Easter Sunday, I hiked around the park in shorts and a T-shirt, only to be snowed on that evening.

While it may seem like blasphemy to inveterate tent campers, I have learned that age (and a bad back) is oft accompanied by an appreciation for indoor plumbing, a proper bed, and a hard roof, underneath which rain can actually be enjoyed. Be sure to check out this park's multibed-room lodge.

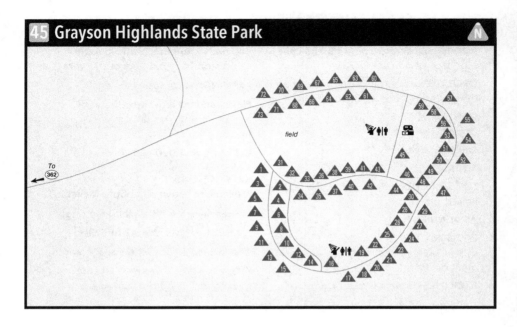

## :: Getting There

From I-81, take Exit 45 at Marion, and drive 33 miles south on VA 16. Turn right onto US 58 in the community of Volney, and continue 8 miles to the park's entrance.

**GPS COORDINATES**  N36° 36.832  W81° 28.860

# 46

# High Knob Recreation Area

*You'll want to make the 1.5-mile (one-way) trek to the observation tower at High Knob.*

**W**ith its small size, seclusion, absence of RV hookups, and small swimming hole located off by itself in the Clinch Ranger District of the George Washington and Jefferson National Forests, remote High Knob Recreation Area is one of those amazing finds that you'll almost want to keep to yourself. But tell your friends—you wouldn't want to deprive them of the magnificent views from the lookout tower.

From the park entrance, it is a 1.7-mile drive down to the day-use section. This area can be lush with hemlocks, rhododendrons, and an understory of ferns, even when the rest of Virginia suffers from drought. Just before the driveway's end on the right side of the road is the trail leading to the High Knob Observation Tower. At the bottom of the driveway is the parking lot for the day-use area and lake on the left. The campground is located to the right and features 13 sites. Because of the narrow, twisty roads leading up to and into the campground, you're not likely to be rubbing elbows with RVers, although RVs of up to 16 feet are welcome.

## :: Ratings

BEAUTY: ★ ★ ★ ★
SITE PRIVACY: ★ ★ ★ ★
SPACIOUSNESS: ★ ★ ★ ★
QUIET: ★ ★ ★ ★ ★
SECURITY: ★ ★ ★
CLEANLINESS: ★ ★ ★ ★ ★

Located at an elevation of 3,800 feet, the 300-foot beach and 4-acre "cold-water" spring-fed lake are guaranteed to provide a refreshing, if not shocking, wake-up call or a pleasant dip on a hot summer afternoon. The ambient temperature in this region can be as much as 20° cooler than the rest of Virginia, which campers appreciate during languid 100°-plus heat waves. The log and stone construction on display at the large bathhouse is the handiwork of CCC workers in the 1930s.

Aside from camping, picnicking, cool bathing, and enjoying the quiet, you'll want to make the 1.5-mile (one-way) trek to the observation tower at High Knob. At an elevation of 4,160 feet, the tower rises 400 feet above the campground and offers outstanding views of five states: Virginia, Kentucky, West Virginia, North Carolina, and Tennessee. Kentucky surface mining can also be seen. This is one of the highest points in Virginia and makes a great spot from which to observe the annual migration of birds of prey in the fall. Nonhikers enjoy this view as well by driving to the tower via FDR 238, but they'll still have to hike a quarter mile to the tower.

The observation tower marks the beginning of the 18.7-mile (point-to-point) Chief Benge Scout Trail, which also wanders past Bark Lake Recreation Area before ending at the Little Stony National Recreation Trail. The Little Stony is a breathtaking

## :: Key Information

**ADDRESS:** Clinch Ranger District, 9416 Darden Ave., Wise, VA 24293

**OPERATED BY:** U.S. Forest Service

**CONTACT:** 276-328-2931; www.fs.usda.gov/activity/gwj /recreation/camping-cabins

**OPEN:** May 15–Sept. 15

**SITES:** 13

**SITE AMENITIES:** Picnic table, fire grill, lantern pole

**ASSIGNMENT:** First come, first served; no reservations

**REGISTRATION:** Self-registration on site

**FACILITIES:** Hot showers, water, flush toilets

**PARKING:** At campsites and day-use area

**FEE:** $10 per night

**ELEVATION:** 3,800 feet

**RESTRICTIONS:**

■ **Pets:** On leash only; not allowed in swimming areas

■ **Fires:** In fire rings, stoves, or grills only

■ **Alcohol:** Prohibited

■ **Vehicles:** Up to 16 feet

■ **Other:** Do not carve, chop, or damage any live trees; keep noise at a reasonable level.

2.8-mile (one-way) trail that follows a former narrow-gauge railroad bed along Little Stony Creek via a 400-foot-deep gorge. Typical of former railroad beds, the Little Stony Trail retains less than a 4% grade. There is some good trout fishing along the Chief Benge Scout Trail, which was built as a joint venture between the Lonesome Pine District of the Boy Scouts and the Clinch Ranger District. Its length belies its level of difficulty, so don't try to cover the 18.7 miles unless you're a seasoned hiker. A more moderate day hike is the 10.5-mile (one-way) walk to Bark Camp Lake, which can be done with a shuttle at the end or as an introductory backpacking outing. Mountain bikers may want to test their mettle on the aforementioned trails, but most of us will enjoy pedaling along the myriad open and gated Forest Service roads that lace the area. Before undertaking any exploration, be sure to pick up a copy of the Clinch Ranger District map from the national forest headquarters in Wise.

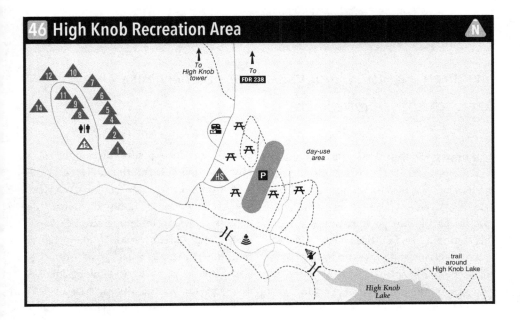

## :: Getting There

From Norton, go 3.7 miles south on VA 619. Turn left onto FDR 238, and follow it 1.6 miles to the campground entrance.

**GPS COORDINATES**   N36° 53.389  W82° 37.330

# 47

# Hungry Mother State Park

*Swimming, boating, and fishing for northern pike are just a few of the possibilities here.*

**H**ungry Mother State Park is one of the original six parks that formed the nucleus of Virginia's state system in 1936. The legend behind this park's name is as colorful as the foliage that wraps around this setting in the fall. Back when relations between settlers and American Indians were at an ebb, it is said that a party of Indian warriors destroyed several settlements south of what is now the park on the New River. Molly Marley and her child escaped the attacks but were taken captive. They eventually escaped, subsisting on wild berries as they made their way through the wilderness. Molly finally collapsed, while her child continued by following a creek. When the child found help, its only words were "hungry, mother." The search party followed the creek and found Molly dead at the base of a mountain. The mountain became Molly's Knob, and the creek was named Hungry Mother Creek. The creek was dammed in 1930 to form Hungry Mother Lake.

The park is located 4 miles from Marion on VA 16, which passes through the park

## :: Ratings

BEAUTY: ★ ★ ★ ★
SITE PRIVACY: ★ ★ ★ ★
SPACIOUSNESS: ★ ★ ★ ★
QUIET: ★ ★ ★ ★
SECURITY: ★ ★ ★
CLEANLINESS: ★ ★ ★ ★

boundaries. Its 94 sites distributed over four campgrounds run the gamut from the 52 newest ones with full hookups (electric, water, and sewer) at Camp Burson to the 11 tents-only sites in campground C. You'll pass Camp Burson on the right prior to reaching Hungry Mother's park entrance. Campground A is located alongside VA 16. This campground sits on a small field with no vegetation between sites and offers little in the way of atmosphere, privacy, or seclusion. Campground B is located across VA 348 and is RV oriented. Its 21 sites have electric and water hookups and are situated close to each other along a maze of hard-surface roads.

Campground C is situated on a neighboring wooded hilltop and will be the likely destination at Hungry Mother for tent camping purists. Park designers utilized this uneven surface by erecting unusual wooden decking for tent pads for most of the sites along this single loop. These sites are interspersed among a forest of oaks and immature pines with some vegetation between them. The positioning of the "tent decks" in terms of location and elevation offers the camper a modicum of privacy at campground C. Sites 4 and 8 offer gravel tent pads rather than decking, and sites 8–11 offer the greatest distance between campers.

Swimming, boating, and fishing for northern pike—reputed to be the best in the state—in the 108-acre Hungry Mother Lake

## :: Key Information

**ADDRESS:** 2854 Park Boulevard, Marion, VA 24354

**OPERATED BY:** Virginia Department of Conservation and Recreation

**CONTACT:** 276-781-7400; virginiastateparks.gov

**OPEN:** First weekend in March–December 1

**SITES:** 94; 11 are designated for tents only

**SITE AMENITIES:** Picnic table, fire grill

**ASSIGNMENT:** First come, first served

**REGISTRATION:** Call 800-933-PARK or visit reserveamerica.com; site assignment on arrival

**FACILITIES:** Cabin rental, fishing, boating, restaurant, flush toilets, showers, pay phone, lake swimming Memorial Day–Labor Day

**PARKING:** 1 vehicle in addition to camping unit at site

**FEE:** Standard tent site $20 per night; $27 per night with electric/water hookups

**ELEVATION:** 2,400 feet

**RESTRICTIONS:**

■ **Pets:** Must be on short leash and attended; $3 per night

■ **Fires:** Use camp stove or fire ring

■ **Alcohol:** Public use or display is prohibited

■ **Vehicles:** Up to 35 feet

■ **Other:** Maximum stay is 14 days in a 30-day period; no cutting live trees; no bringing firewood into park so as not to introduce wood-boring insects; maximum 6 people per site; quiet hours 10 p.m.–6 a.m.; gasoline motors not allowed on lake

are but a few of the activities at the park. The fishing pier is wheelchair accessible. This 2,215-acre getaway offers approximately 12 miles of trails for hiking and biking. Bicycles are allowed on the 2.9-mile Lake Trail, 1-mile Powder House Trail, 1-mile Old Shawnee Trail, 1.2-mile Fisherman's Run Trail, and 0.9-mile Raider's Run Trail. Hungry Mother also has the distinction of being the only Virginia state park with a conference center. Hemlock Haven's meeting rooms hold 10–375 people.

Hungry Mother offers interpretive programming throughout the summer, including an arts and crafts festival in July and the Mountain Do Triathlon in late April. Occurring on a more regular basis are canoe tours, night hikes, campfires, music in the amphitheater, lectures, and activity workshops. Past workshops have included bat house building, live snake viewing, Appalachian toy construction, and bird feeder building. Wee Naturalist and Junior Naturalist programs occur once or twice a week to teach kids about the outdoors and environmental conservation. In short, there is plenty going on at Hungry Mother State Park for the entire family.

While it may seem like blasphemy to inveterate tent campers, I have learned that age (and a bad back) is oft accompanied by an appreciation for indoor plumbing, a proper bed, and a hard roof, underneath which rain can actually be enjoyed. Be sure to check out this park's array of cabins and its multibedroom lodge.

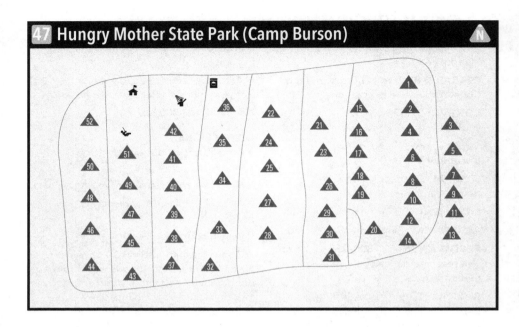

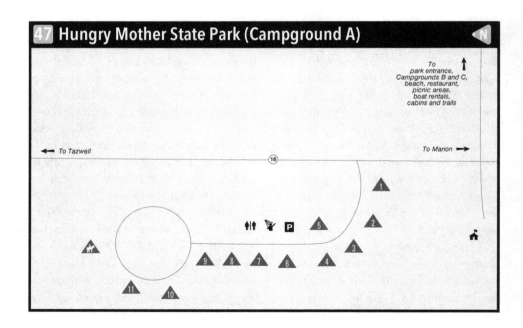

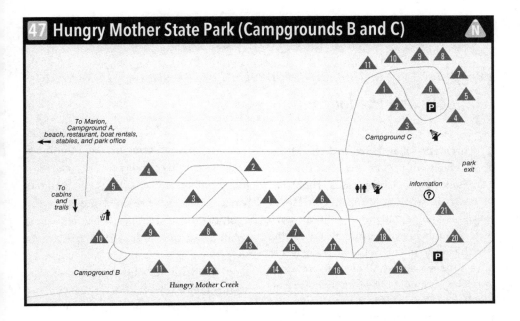

**47 Hungry Mother State Park (Campgrounds B and C)**

To Marion,
Campground A,
beach, restaurant, boat rentals,
← stables, and park office

Campground C

To
cabins
and
trails ↓

park
exit

information

Campground B

*Hungry Mother Creek*

## :: Getting There

From I-81, take Exit 47 heading toward Marion on US 11. Turn right in Marion onto VA 16, and continue 4 miles to the park's entrance.

**GPS COORDINATES**   N36° 53.428  W81° 31.208

# 48

# Hurricane Campground

*Few places rival this setting, nestled in the shade of towering hemlocks and rhododendrons.*

**H**urricane **Campground** is ideally located with good access to the Iron Mountain, Appalachian, and Highlands Horse Trails and in close proximity to Mount Rogers—Virginia's highest point at 5,729 feet. Mount Rogers National Recreation Area has an abundance of campgrounds that attract many visitors. All of them are excellent campgrounds, but given a choice, follow Robert Frost's lead—take a chance and pitch a tent at the campground less visited.

Hurricane Campground is off VA 16, south of Marion. Quite a few sites are located along the creek. The first site on the right is arguably one of the best campsites anywhere. Few campsites rival this setting—it's well off the campground road, out of sight from any other campsites, bordered by a pleasant stream and nestled in the shade of towering hemlocks and rhododendrons. All of the campsites at Hurricane Campground offer more than a modicum of privacy and solitude. Be sure to look around before picking a site and pitching your tent, as individual tastes may vary.

## :: Ratings

BEAUTY: ★ ★ ★ ★
SITE PRIVACY: ★ ★ ★ ★
SPACIOUSNESS: ★ ★ ★ ★ ★
QUIET: ★ ★ ★ ★
SECURITY: ★ ★ ★
CLEANLINESS: ★ ★ ★

The paved campground continues straight, running parallel to the creek with sites 12, 18, 19, and 20 sitting right along its banks. Once you've reached site 20 on the right, the road curves to the left and winds uphill along the flank of Hurricane Knob. Sites 22–26 offer seclusion and could be good choices when the streams are overflowing their banks. Site 26 is situated at the end of the campground loop and offers the additional benefit of limited drive-by traffic.

As its name suggests, Mount Rogers National Recreation Area is geared toward recreation. In addition to its seclusion, Hurricane Campground provides an excellent base camp from which to explore some outstanding trails and forest roads by foot, horse, or mountain bike.

The trailhead for the 1-mile Hurricane Knob Loop Trail is located at the entrance to the campground across from the information kiosk. The 9.6-mile Four Trails Circuit covers bits of the Dickey Knob, Comers Creek Falls, Iron Mountain, and Appalachian Trails as it winds its way through some of the Mount Rogers NRA's finest woodland scenery. For that matter, you can pick up a national forest map and plan to walk a given distance on either the Iron Mountain or Appalachian Trail, both of which are ubiquitous in this 115,000-acre recreation area. Sixty miles of AT carve their way through the Mount Rogers area.

## :: Key Information

**ADDRESS:** Mount Rogers National Recreation Area, 2021 Hurricane Campground Road, Sugar Grove, VA 24375

**OPERATED BY:** U.S. Forest Service

**CONTACT:** 276-783-5196; www.fs.usda.gov/gwj

**OPEN:** April–October

**SITES:** 26

**SITE AMENITIES:** Picnic table, fire grill, lantern pole

**ASSIGNMENT:** First come, first served; reservations at recreation.gov or 877-444-6777

**REGISTRATION:** On site

**FACILITIES:** Flush toilets, warm showers

**PARKING:** At campsite

**FEE:** Single $16 per night; double $32 per night

**ELEVATION:** 2,880 feet

**RESTRICTIONS:**
- **Pets:** Must be on leash and attended
- **Fires:** Use available grills
- **Alcohol:** Prohibited
- **Vehicles:** Up to 22 feet
- **Other:** Maximum stay is 21 days in a 30-day period; no cutting live trees; quiet time 10 p.m.–6 a.m.

Mountain bikes are not allowed on the Appalachian Trail or in federally designated Wilderness areas; otherwise, possibilities for two-wheel fun seem limitless. Back when the sport was still new to Virginia and other park agencies were not aware of its existence, the folks in this district of the Jefferson National Forest were bold enough to proclaim that "whoever invented mountain bicycles surely had the Mount Rogers National Recreation Area in mind!" Those looking for minimal challenge and maximum fun will head for the 33-mile (one-way) Virginia Creeper Trail, a converted railroad bed that runs downhill from Whitetop Mountain to the town of Damascus. The Iron Mountain Trail gets a lot of use from local mountain bikers, as well as visitors looking for additional technical and aerobic challenges. Combine sections of the Iron Mountain Trail with gravel Forest Service roads to create your own loop, or pick up one of the several guides that detail tried-and-true loop rides. Sections of the orange-blazed Virginia Highlands Horse Trail are also open to bikers, but be sure to yield the right-of-way to equestrians. If trout fishing is your passion, then look no further than Hurricane Creek or Comers Creek. Angling opportunities abound on more than 100 miles of streams and two lakes within the area.

Mount Rogers NRA has no shortage of superb camping destinations. In addition to those detailed in this book, there are the Beartree Recreation Area (90 sites), Grindstone Recreation Area (108 sites), Raccoon Branch Campground (20 sites), Stony Fork Campground (54 sites), and Fox Creek Horse Campground (32 sites). You can get additional information at **www.fs.usda.gov/gwj**. Once you arrive, be sure to stop by the Mount Rogers ranger station on VA 16 for a district map and trail brochures. When a national forest district has the word "recreation" in its name, you can be sure that camping accommodations and outdoor activities will be awesome.

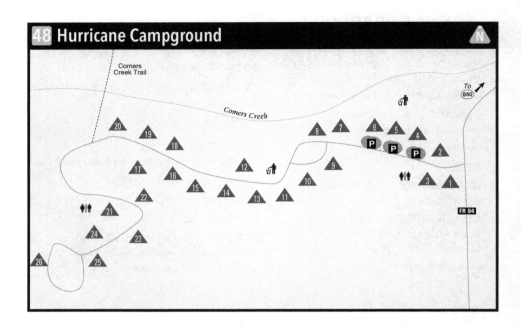

## :: Getting There

From I-81, take Exit 45 onto VA 16 south, and drive 15 miles. After entering the Mount Rogers NRA, turn right onto VA 650 and continue 2 miles to the entrance to Hurricane Campground.

**GPS COORDINATES**   N36° 43.330  W81° 29.267

# 49

# Natural Tunnel State Park

*Natural Tunnel was dubbed the Eighth Wonder of the World by former Secretary of State William Jennings Bryan.*

**N**atural **Tunnel State Park** offers glimpses into both historic and pre-historic periods. The tunnel itself formed as the result of groundwater containing carbonic acid seeping through and dissolving massive limestone deposits to create a cave that grew to 850 feet in length and 100 feet in height with the assistance of some blasting. Fossils can be seen along the bed of Stock Creek, which traverses the tunnel, as well as on the tunnel walls. Former Secretary of State William Jennings Bryan called Natural Tunnel the Eighth Wonder of the World, and visitors have been flocking here for more than 100 years. Because of its location in the shadow of the Cumberland Gap, through which the country's earliest settlers crossed on their westward passage, it should come as little surprise that Daniel Boone is thought to have been one of the first Europeans to view this natural wonder. But it was not written about until Col. Stephen Long did so in the March 1832 *Monthly American Journal of Geology and Natural Science*. Final blasting was done to open both ends of the tunnel to allow for the South Atlantic and Ohio Railroad to lay down tracks and pass through, and coal trains continue to do so.

This 950-acre park has two campgrounds, along with 10 two- to three-bedroom cabins that can be rented. After driving uphill on the park road, you will first pass Cove View Campground, the older of the two campgrounds. It includes 16 sites, all of which include electric and water hookups. Sites are laid out on a large grassy field that is crisscrossed by short gravel roads. The campground is fairly open, providing little in the way of privacy between sites. However, the advantage is that these sites are all pull-through, making life a little easier for those pulling a camper trailer. Tent campers will probably want to find a site across the park road in the Lovers Leap Campground, which is surrounded by thick vegetation. At first glance, these 18 sites with their gravel surfaces appear more RV oriented, but a closer look reveals that each has a 15-foot-square finer gravel tent pad. Sites are laid out along a small loop, but I found that interior sites 15–18 offer the most privacy. These few campsites are elevated from the outer loop and include some desirable shrubbery between sites, including blackberry bushes.

Campground activities could include swimming in the Junior Olympic pool, hiking or biking on the park's trail system,

## :: Ratings

BEAUTY: ★ ★ ★
SITE PRIVACY: ★ ★
SPACIOUSNESS: ★ ★ ★
QUIET: ★ ★
SECURITY: ★ ★
CLEANLINESS: ★ ★ ★ ★

## :: Key Information

**ADDRESS:** 1420 Natural Tunnel Parkway, Duffield, VA 24244

**OPERATED BY:** Virginia Department of Conservation and Recreation

**CONTACT:** 276-940-2674; dcr.virginia.gov

**OPEN:** March 1–early December

**SITES:** 34

**SITE AMENITIES:** Picnic table, fire ring, lantern pole, electric/water hookups

**ASSIGNMENT:** First come, first served

**REGISTRATION:** Call 800-933-PARK or visit reserveamerica.com, or on arrival; reservations highly recommended

**FACILITIES:** Water, hot showers, laundry, camp store, pay phone

**PARKING:** 2 vehicles per site in addition to camping unit

**FEE:** $27 per night, plus $5 transaction fee for each transaction

**ELEVATION:** 1,400 feet

**RESTRICTIONS:**
▪ **Pets:** On leash or in enclosed area
▪ **Fires:** In fire rings, stoves, or grills only
▪ **Alcohol:** Prohibited
▪ **Vehicles:** Up to 34 feet
▪ **Other:** Do not damage any trees; quiet hours 10 p.m.–6 a.m.

and playing horseshoes. Unique to Natural Tunnel State Park is a 12-minute chairlift that begins at the visitor center and drops 200 feet to the tunnel opening.

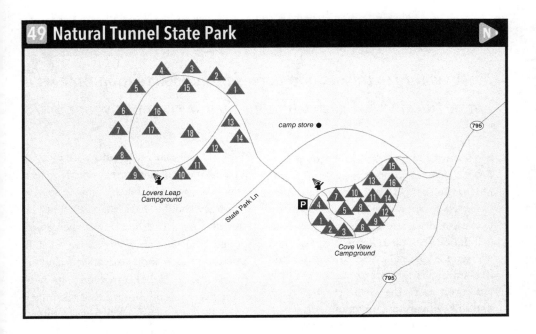

## :: Getting There

Natural Tunnel State Park is in Scott County, about 13 miles north of Gate City and 20 miles north of Kingsport, TN. From I-81, take US 23 north to Gate City (about 20 miles). The turnoff to the park is at mile marker 17.4 on US 23. Take Natural Tunnel Parkway about 1 mile east to the park entrance.

**GPS COORDINATES**  N36° 42.389 W82° 44.270

# 50

# Raven Cliff Campground

*Most visitors to this 115,000-acre National Recreation Area will not be flocking to Raven Cliff. But their oversight is your gain.*

**R**aven Cliff is farther from Mount Rogers than any other campground in the Mount Rogers National Recreation Area. Given its location and absence of amenities, most visitors to this 119,000-acre NRA will not be flocking to Raven Cliff. But their oversight is your gain. The agricultural land that surrounds the campground gives little indication as to the environmental niche that this campground occupies.

After passing through a flat, open area consistent with the rural surroundings, you'll enter a narrow ravine through which Cripple Creek (of the famed bluegrass tune) passes. A steep cliff lines the creek on one side, while a grassy open area for equestrian campers is on the other. This free-flowing trout waterway creates a beautiful scene as it courses through this gorge.

The campground loop is located across the road from the covered picnic pavilion just up from the entrance. Turn left into the campground, and you'll find 20 sites (14/15 is a double site) tucked onto the side of Gleaves Knob under a canopy of pine,

hemlock, and oak. Sites 1 and 2 are located at the near end of the campground loop just outside the gated entrance. Those in search of privacy should check the availability of sites 18–20 at the other end of the campground road. Site 20 is located on a small turnaround loop and is the most secluded. This is a great little campground. Its out-of-the-way location minimizes the number of campers, its lush trees help keep things quiet, and its out-and-back road past the 20 sites limits drive-through traffic. If you don't mind driving to reach the Iron Mountain Trail, Appalachian Trail, Virginia Creeper Trail, and others in the Mount Rogers Recreation Area—or you're just looking for a great, secluded campground at which to pitch your tent—then Raven Cliff could be the place for your next camping trip.

However, Mount Rogers NRA has no shortage of superb camping destinations. In addition to those detailed in this book, there are also the Beartree Recreation Area (90 sites), Grindstone Recreation Area (108 sites), Raccoon Branch Campground (20 sites), Stony Fork Campground (54 sites), and Fox Creek Horse Campground (32 sites). You can get additional information at **www.fs.usda.gov/gwj**. Once you arrive, be sure to stop at the Mount Rogers ranger station on VA 16 for a district map and trail brochures. When a national forest district has the word "recreation" in its name, you can

## :: Ratings

BEAUTY: ★ ★ ★ ★
SITE PRIVACY: ★ ★ ★ ★
SPACIOUSNESS: ★ ★ ★ ★ ★
QUIET: ★ ★ ★ ★ ★
SECURITY: ★ ★ ★
CLEANLINESS: ★ ★ ★

# :: Key Information

**ADDRESS:** Mount Rogers National Recreation Area, 544 Raven Cliff Lane, Ivanhoe, VA 24350

**OPERATED BY:** U.S. Forest Service

**CONTACT:** www.fs.usda.gov/gwj

**OPEN:** April 15–Oct. 31

**SITES:** 20

**SITE AMENITIES:** Picnic table, fire grill, lantern pole

**ASSIGNMENT:** First come, first served

**REGISTRATION:** On site

**FACILITIES:** Vault toilet, water

**PARKING:** At campsite and day-use area

**FEE:** $5 per night

**ELEVATION:** 2,240 feet

**RESTRICTIONS:**
- **Pets:** Must be on leash and attended
- **Fires:** Use camp stove or fire ring
- **Alcohol:** Prohibited
- **Vehicles:** Up to 32 feet
- **Other:** Maximum stay is 21 days in a 30-day period; Forest Service does not plow snow; no cutting live trees; quiet time 10 p.m.–6 a.m.

be sure that camping accommodations and outdoor activities will be awesome.

Take the 1-mile (out-and-back) walk along Cripple Creek on the Raven Cliff Furnace Trail to see the remains of the furnace, in use until the early 1900s. Iron ore was mixed with limestone and charcoal and combined under extreme temperatures to form "pigs," which were then shipped to Richmond and other sites for casting.

While Raven Cliff is far from the various trails and recreational attractions that the Mount Rogers NRA has to offer, mountain bikers enjoy a degree of comfort from Raven Cliff's relative proximity to the 57-mile New River State Park. Head south on VA 94, and turn left on VA 602 to get on the trail at the Byllesby Dam. The dam is near the southwestern prongs of the trail, which end at Fries (pronounced "freeze") and Galax. Heading northeast on this converted railroad bed will also have you pedaling downhill for the better

part of 30 miles toward the trail's northeastern terminus at Pulaski. The last 10 miles from Draper to Pulaski are on a slight uphill slope. In addition to largely avoiding vehicular traffic, one of the great advantages of rail-to-trail conversions such as the New River Trail is the modest gradient. The downhills are enjoyable, and the uphills are very bearable.

Pedaling along this slight incline on the well-graded cinder surface is probably the easiest riding you're going to do. If you're planning an out-and-back, however, and a 60-miler sounds too ambitious, pedal from the Byllesby Dam at mile 37.3 to Shot Tower State Park at mile 25.2 along the New River Trail. This is a manageable 24-mile round-trip. In addition to safe and pleasant conditions on the trail, the scenery along this river—thought to be the oldest in North America—is outstanding. Raven Cliff's proximity to the New River opens up possibilities for paddlers and anglers too.

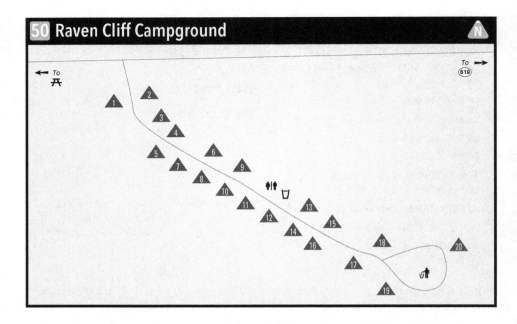

## :: Getting There

From Wytheville, take US 21 to the community of Speedwell. Turn left onto VA 619 and drive 6.5 miles to the campground entrance on the right.

**GPS COORDINATES**   N36° 50.159  W81° 03.928

# APPENDIX A

## Camping Equipment Checklist

I keep a plastic storage container full of the essentials of car camping (except for the large and bulky items on this list) so that they're ready to go when I am. I make a last-minute check of the inventory, resupply anything that's low or missing, and away I go!

### COOKING UTENSILS

Bottle opener

Bottles of salt, pepper, spices, sugar, cooking oil, and maple syrup in waterproof, spill-proof containers

Can opener

Corkscrew

Cups, plastic or tin

Dish soap *(biodegradable)*, sponge, and towel

Flatware

Food of your choice

Frying pan

Fuel for stove

Matches in waterproof container

Plates

Pocketknife

Pot with lid

Spatula

Stove

Tinfoil

Wooden spoon

### FIRST AID KIT

Band-Aids

First aid cream

Gauze pads

Ibuprofen or aspirin

Insect repellent

Moleskin

Snakebite kit (if you're heading for desert conditions)

Sunscreen/lip balm

Tape, waterproof adhesive

### SLEEPING GEAR

Pillow

Sleeping bag

Sleeping pad, inflatable or insulated

Tent with ground tarp and rainfly

### MISCELLANEOUS

Bath soap *(biodegradable)*, washcloth, and towel

Camp chair

Candles

Cooler

Deck of cards

Fire starter

Flashlight with fresh batteries

Foul-weather clothing

Paper towels

Plastic zip-top bags

Sunglasses

Toilet paper

Water bottle

Wool blanket

### OPTIONAL

Barbecue grill

Binoculars

Books on bird, plant, and wildlife identification

Fishing rod and tackle

Hatchet

Lantern

Maps *(road, topographic, trail, etc.)*

# APPENDIX B

• • • • • • • • • • • • • • • • • • • • • • •

## Sources of Information

The following is a partial list of agencies, associations, and organizations to write or call for information on outdoor recreation opportunities in Virginia.

**BLUE RIDGE PARKWAY**
199 Hemphill Knob Road
Asheville, NC 28803
(828) 298-0398
**nps.gov/blri**

**GEORGE WASHINGTON AND JEFFERSON NATIONAL FORESTS**
5162 Valleypointe Parkway
Roanoke, VA 24019
(540) 265-5100
**www.fs.usda.gov/gwj**

**SHENANDOAH NATIONAL PARK**
3655 U.S. Highway 211 E.
Luray, VA 22835
(540) 999-3500
**nps.gov/shen**

**VIRGINIA DEPARTMENT OF CONSERVATION AND RECREATION**
203 Governor Street, Ste. 213
Richmond, VA 23219
(800) 933-park
**dcr.virginia.gov/state_parks**

**VIRGINIA DEPARTMENT OF GAME AND INLAND FISHERIES**
4010 W. Broad Street
Richmond, VA 23230
(804) 367-1000
**www.dgif.virginia.gov**

# APPENDIX C

● ● ● ● ● ● ● ● ● ● ● ● ● ● ● ● ● ● ● ● ●

## Suggested Reading and Reference

*The Best of the Appalachian Trail Overnight Hikes.* Logue, Victoria and Frank. Adkins, Leonard M. Menasha Ridge Press, 2007.

*The Best of the Appalachian Trail Day Hikes.* Logue, Victoria and Frank. Adkins, Leonard M. Menasha Ridge Press, 2004.

*Civil War Virginia: Battleground for a Nation.* Robertson, James I. University Press of Virginia, 1993.

*Day and Overnight Hikes in the Shenandoah National Park.* Molloy, Johnny. Menasha Ridge Press, 2007.

*Highroad Guide to the Virginia Mountains.* Winegar, Deane and Garvey. Longstreet Press, 2003.

*Mountain Bike! Virginia.* Porter, Randy. Menasha Ridge Press, 2001.

*Notes on the State of Virginia.* Jefferson, Thomas. W.W. Norton & Company, 1998.

*Roadside Geology of Virginia.* Frye, Keith. Mountain Press Publishing Company, 2003.

*Shenandoah National Park: An Interpretive Guide.* Conners, James A. The McDonald & Woodward Publishing Company, 1988.

*Virginia: A Guide to Backcountry Travel & Adventure.* Bannon, James. Out There Press, 1997.

# INDEX

# ABOUT THE AUTHOR

**R**andy Porter resides in a cabin in the woods at the foot of the Blue Ridge Mountains west of Charlottesville, Virginia. His travels throughout Virginia have covered most every corner over the past 40 years, but he's now largely content to remain closer to home, relishing the wildlife that comes to his windows and reliving vicariously through the adventures of his 20-something-year-old son, Chris.

**DEAR CUSTOMERS AND FRIENDS,**

**SUPPORTING YOUR INTEREST IN OUTDOOR ADVENTURE,** travel, and an active lifestyle is central to our operations, from the authors we choose to the locations we detail to the way we design our books. Menasha Ridge Press was incorporated in 1982 by a group of veteran outdoorsmen and professional outfitters. For many years now, we've specialized in creating books that benefit the outdoors enthusiast.

Almost immediately, Menasha Ridge Press earned a reputation for revolutionizing outdoors- and travel-guidebook publishing. For such activities as canoeing, kayaking, hiking, backpacking, and mountain biking, we established new standards of quality that transformed the whole genre, resulting in outdoor-recreation guides of great sophistication and solid content. Menasha Ridge continues to be outdoor publishing's greatest innovator.

The folks at Menasha Ridge Press are as at home on a white-water river or mountain trail as they are editing a manuscript. The books we build for you are the best they can be, because we're responding to your needs. Plus, we use and depend on them ourselves.

We look forward to seeing you on the river or the trail. If you'd like to contact us directly, join in at www.trekalong.com or visit us at www.menasharidge.com. We thank you for your interest in our books and the natural world around us all.

**SAFE TRAVELS,**

**BOB SEHLINGER**
**PUBLISHER**

FEB 0 1 2019

CPSIA information can be obtained
at www.ICGtesting.com
Printed in the USA
LVHW08*1628111018
593268LV00011B/227/P

9 781634 042048